Optical Coherence Tomography

Aniz Girach • Robert C. Sergott

Editors

Optical Coherence Tomography

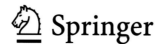

Editors
Aniz Girach
London
UK

Robert C. Sergott
Neuro-Ophthalmology Service
Wills Eye Institute
Philadelphia
Pennsylvania
USA

ISBN 978-3-319-24815-8   ISBN 978-3-319-24817-2   (eBook)
DOI 10.1007/978-3-319-24817-2

Library of Congress Control Number: 2015959795

Springer Cham Heidelberg New York Dordrecht London

Printed on acid-free paper

Springer International Publishing AG Switzerland is part of Springer Science+Business Media (www.springer.com)

Preface

The eye is a miraculous structure with inherent self-healing properties. Yet, nature has a way of interfering with this process, causing disease. None is more devastating than the occurrence of retinal diseases or retinal manifestations of non-retinal ocular disease. If the disease is on the surface of the retina and has gross pathology, then this can be visualised easily with available techniques. However, the challenge remains in visualising microscopic pathology of the surface or different layers of the retina. In these circumstances, conventional diagnostic techniques to help diagnose and manage patients adequately have failed ophthalmologists over the years. There was a clear need for more detailed imaging technology of the retina. Optical coherence tomography (OCT) has paved this way and changed the whole paradigm of visualisation of the retina.

OCT has revolutionised the diagnosis and management of patients with retinal and non-retinal diseases. OCT has gone through various phases of development, and modern methods outlined in this book are the latest technological breakthroughs in the field.

This book contains contributions from an internationally renowned group of experts from the field of ophthalmology and ophthalmic imaging. The initial chapter covers the basic principles and interpretation of OCT. This is followed by chapters covering the various key retinal diseases and their diagnosis and management. A key feature of this book was to also include chapters on other diseases such as glaucoma, uveitis and optic disc disease, as well as covering topics such as toxic or nutritional conditions and other hot topics leading to retinal disease. The book contains a plethora of clinical case reports supplemented by OCT images utilising the latest in imaging technology.

It is hoped that this book, with its emphasis on clinical ophthalmology, will provide educational material to a wide ranging audience—from the medical student, optometrist, resident or fellow who is eager to learn about the latest techniques being employed in the clinic to the practising ophthalmologist who can utilise the plentiful case reports and images to educate him-/ herself.

London, UK   Aniz Girach, MBChB, MRCGP, MRCOphth, MD

Philadelphia, PA, USA   Bob Sergott, MD

Abbreviations

ARMD	Age-related macular degeneration
APMPPE	Acute posterior multifocal placoid pigment epitheliopathy
AZOOR	Acute zonal occult outer retinopathy
BCVA	Best corrected visual acuity
BRAO	Branch retinal artery occlusion
BRVO	Branch retinal vein occlusion
CIS	Clinically isolated syndrome
CRION	Chronic relapsing inflammatory optic neuritis
CRVO	Central retinal vein occlusion
DME	Diabetic macular edema
DUSN	Diffuse unilateral subacute neuroretinitis
EDI-OCT	Enhanced depth imaging OCT
ERM	Epiretinal membrane
FA	Fluorescein angiogram
FEVR	Familial exudative vitreoretinopathy
GA	Geographic atrophy
HRVO	Hemi-retinal vein occlusion
HVF	Humphrey visual fields
ICG	Indocyanine green angiography
IgG	Immunoglobulin G
IIH	Idiopathic intracranial hypertension
ILM	Internal limiting membrane
IN	OCT International Nomenclature for Optical Coherence Tomography
IS/OS	Inner segment/outer segment
IRVAN	Idiopathic retinal vasculitis, aneurysms and neuroretinitis syndrome
IUSG	International Uveitis Study Group
IVTH	International Vitreomacular Traction Study
MEWDS	Multiple evanescent white dot syndrome
MDR-TB	Multidrug-resistant tuberculosis
MFS	Multifocal choroiditis with panuveitis
MRI	Magnetic resonance imaging
MRV	Magnetic resonance venography
MRSA	Methicillin-resistant *Staphylococcus aureus*
MS	Multiple sclerosis
NAION	Non-arteritic ischemic optic neuropathy

NMO	Neuromyelitis optica
OCT	Optical coherence tomography
OD	Oculus dexter
ONHD	Optic nerve head drusen
OS	Oculus sinister
PED	Pigment epithelial detachments
PIC	Punctate inner choroiditis
PFT	Parafoveal telangiectasia
PRP	Panretinal photocoagulation
RAM	Retinal arterial macroaneurysm
RNFL	Retinal nerve fibre layer
ROP	Retinopathy of prematurity
RPE	Retinal pigment epithelium
RRMS	Relapsing-remitting multiple sclerosis
SD-OCT	Spectral domain OCT
SHYPS	Subretinal hyporeflective space
SUN	Standardization of Uveitis Nomenclature
TAA	Tobacco alcohol amblyopia
TRD	Tractional retinal detachment
VEGF	Vascular endothelial growth factor

Contents

Contributors

Aniz Girach, MD Chief Medical Officer, Nightstarx, Wellcome Trust, London, UK

Craig M. Greven, MD Department of Ophthalmology, Wills Eye Hospital, Philadelphia, PA, USA

Margaret A. Greven, MD Department of Ophthalmology, Wills Eye Hospital, Philadelphia, PA, USA

Alexander Juhn, BA Department of Ophthalmology, Wills Eye Hospital, Philadelphia, PA, USA

M. Ali Khan, MD Retina Service, Wills Eye Hospital, Philadelphia, PA, USA

Teri T. Kleinberg, MD, MSc Department of Neuro-Ophthalmology, Wills Eye Hospital, Philadelphia, PA, USA

Joan Lee, DO Department of Ophthalmology, Geisinger Hospital, Danville, PA, USA

David H. Perlmutter, MD Department of Ophthalmology, Wills Eye Hospital, Philadelphia, PA, USA

David A. Salz, MD Department of Ophthalmology, Wills Eye Hospital, Philadelphia, PA, USA

Robert C. Sergott, MD Neuro-Ophthalmology Service, Wills Eye Hospital, Philadelphia, PA, USA

Priya Sharma, MD Department of Ophthalmology, Wills Eye Hospital, Philadelphia, PA, USA

Daniel W. Upton, MD Department of Ophthalmology, Geisinger Medical Center, Danville, PA, USA

Guide to OCT Image Interpretation with Normal and Anatomic Variants

Priya Sharma and Robert C. Sergott

Abstract

Optical coherence tomography (OCT) is a useful adjunct imaging technique for retinal and optic nerve pathology. Advances in OCT have made it a useful diagnostic tool in ethambutol toxicity, hydroxychloroquine retinopathy, optic nerve head drusen, glaucoma, idiopathic intracranial hypertension, and multiple sclerosis, to name a few conditions. Care should be taken when interpreting OCT data, as errors and artifacts can occur. However, OCT has revolutionized ophthalmology and will continue to shape the ophthalmic field as new advances develop.

Keywords

Optical coherence tomography • Normal anatomy • Artifacts • Multicolor • Ethambutol • Hydroxychloroquine • Optic nerve head drusen • Glaucoma • Idiopathic intracranial hypertension • Multiple sclerosis

P. Sharma, MD
Department of Ophthalmology, Wills Eye Hospital, Philadelphia, PA, USA
e-mail: psharma@willseye.org

R.C. Sergott, MD (✉)
Neuro-Ophthalmology Service, Wills Eye Hospital, Philadelphia, PA, USA
e-mail: rcs220@comcast.net

History of Optical Coherence Tomography

Imaging techniques have gained popularity as a useful adjunctive technology to diagnosis and management in ophthalmology. Techniques such as ultrasound imaging, computed tomography, and magnetic resonance imaging have been useful adjuncts, but all are limited for fine intraocular evaluation. However, in 1991, a technique called optical coherence tomography (OCT) was first demonstrated [1] and became commercially available in 1996 (Humphrey Systems, Dublin, CA) [2].

OCT is a noninvasive medical imaging technique that utilizes the principle of optical scattering to reconstruct intraocular images. An optical signal is either transmitted through or reflected by a tissue, and these different signals are used to reconstruct a spatial picture of the tissue being imaged [1].

Advances in OCT technology have quickly transformed it into one of the indispensable techniques for ophthalmology and arguably has transformed it into the most utilized imaging technology. Refinements such as higher acquisition rates of images, higher resolution of images, and increasing ability to image transparent tissues in the anterior segment have been indispensable. Most recently, advances such as swept-source OCT (SS-OCT) and OCT-angiography (OCT-A) have even given the ability to reconstruct an angiographic image and utilize a multilayered assessment to retinal pathology [3]. Another imaging technique, multicolor OCT, has been developed for spectral-domain OCT (SD-OCT, Heidelberg Engineering, Heidelberg, Germany), in which three simultaneously acquired reflective images are created using three laser wavelengths of blue, green, and infrared, as another means of cross-sectional imaging [4].

Normal Anatomy

Advances in resolution of OCT have made ultra-fine structural detail possible. The anatomic correlates have been increasingly speculated, but a recent international committee joined to create a consensus nomenclature for OCT [5].

The consensus nomenclature helps clinicians by defining structures on OCT, therefore making standardized interpretation possible. Starting from the inner retina, the first hyperreflective band that is occasionally evident is the posterior cortical vitreous, and analysis of this line can be helpful for conditions such as posterior vitreous detachment or vitreomacular traction. After this, a hyporeflective preretinal space may be evident. Next, the hyperreflective nerve fiber layer is present, often attenuated in conditions such as glaucomatous optic neuropathy. The next series of alternating hypo- and hyperreflective bands correspond to the consecutive retinal layers, as is seen in Fig. 1.1. Close analysis of these layers can give evidence as to varying pathology. For example, hyperreflective areas in the outer plexiform layer could suggest exudates from diabetic retinopathy, whereas atrophy of the inner retinal layers could suggest a central retinal artery occlusion. Closer to the inner retina, the ellipsoid zone, or the hyperreflective region of the photoreceptor with densely packed mitochondria, has gained scrutiny recently with the advent of ocriplasmin injections and is thought to account for a large part of vision [6, 7]. The ellipsoid zone is also examined in any patient complaining of unexplained visual loss, to see if disruption of the photoreceptors could account for their visual symptoms.

OCT can also be helpful for imaging the choroid, although the choriocapillaris can be imaged with more clarity using enhanced-depth imaging OCT (EDI-OCT) of the choroid.

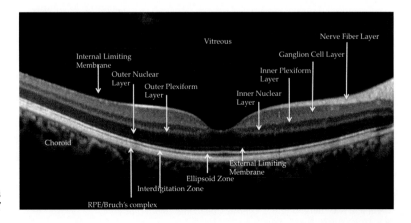

Fig. 1.1 Normal anatomic landmarks as defined by the IN OCT Consensus [5], on a representative patient's OCT

Conditions in Which OCT Is Helpful

Medication Toxicity

Ethambutol

Ethambutol optic neuropathy is a type of toxic optic neuropathy characterized by bilateral, painless vision loss that progresses with continued intake of the medication [8]. Classically, ethambutol-associated optic neuropathy has been monitored with the use of Ishihara pseudoisochromatic color plates, visual field testing, and serial best-corrected visual acuities. However, OCT could be a helpful adjunctive technique, as it can demonstrate early retinal ganglion layer loss with preferential papillomacular bundle loss that may precede other clinical signs of toxic neuropathy [9]. Early detection of ethambutol optic neuropathy can be helpful, as the vision and structural loss are largely reversible in many cases.

Hydroxychloroquine

Hydroxychloroquine is a disease-modifying antirheumatic drug that is used for the chronic treatment of certain rheumatologic and dermatologic conditions. Retinal toxicity remains a well-known side effect of chronic use, with the risk increasing with higher cumulative doses over 1,000 g or daily intake of more than 5–6.5 mg/kg/day. Early detection of retinal toxicity is imperative, as it is often irreversible and can progress even if therapy has been discontinued [10].

The current screening protocol for hydroxychloroquine toxicity includes 10-2 Humphrey Visual Fields (HVFs) along with SD-OCT to detect early perifoveal ellipsoid changes in a "flying saucer sign" [11].

Optic Nerve Head Drusen (ONHD)

The presence of optic disk obscuration on clinical exam can be the initial trigger that leads to an extensive evaluation for optic disk edema, including magnetic resonance imaging (MRI) and magnetic resonance venography (MRV). However, in certain subsets of individuals, the presence of optic nerve head drusen (ONHD) can create the clinical appearance of disk elevation, due to congenital buried foci of calcium. ONHD classically appear on B-scan ultrasonography as hyperreflective elements that persist at low gain, but small-buried ONHD can sometimes be difficult to visualize.

OCT can show optically empty cavities posterior to disk elevation, which correspond to buried drusen. Additionally, OCT visualization of the peripapillary retinal nerve fiber layer (RNFL) with SD-OCT can be useful to differentiate optic disk edema from ONHD [12]. Recent reports have also noted that enhanced-depth imaging OCT (EDI-OCT) and SS-OCT allow better detection of ONHD and help to correlate drusen with associated visual field changes [13].

Glaucoma

Glaucoma is a progressive loss of peripheral nerve fiber layers due to many underlying risk factors, the most well known of which is intraocular pressure. Classically, peripheral visual field loss on HVF has been a sign of glaucoma, and visual field defects are followed over time to detect progression. However, often visual fields are unreliable or change significantly from visit to visit, depending on patient attention and fatiguability. Therefore, OCT can serve as a useful adjunct to follow glaucomatous changes over time in patients who do not test well with HVF [14, 15] (Fig. 1.2).

Idiopathic Intracranial Hypertension

Patients with idiopathic intracranial hypertension (IIH) often present with bilateral optic disk edema from elevated intracranial pressure, which commonly responds to acetazolamide. If responding well to therapy, optic disk edema should decrease or stay stable over time. Classically, response to acetazolamide was measured by serial repeat lumbar punctures to measure opening pressure of the cerebrospinal fluid, to guide titration of acetazolamide along with assessment of the need for surgical intervention. However, with the onset of OCT, quantitative measurements of optic disk edema can help guide response therapy, thereby replacing the need for repeated lumbar punctures [16] (Fig. 1.3).

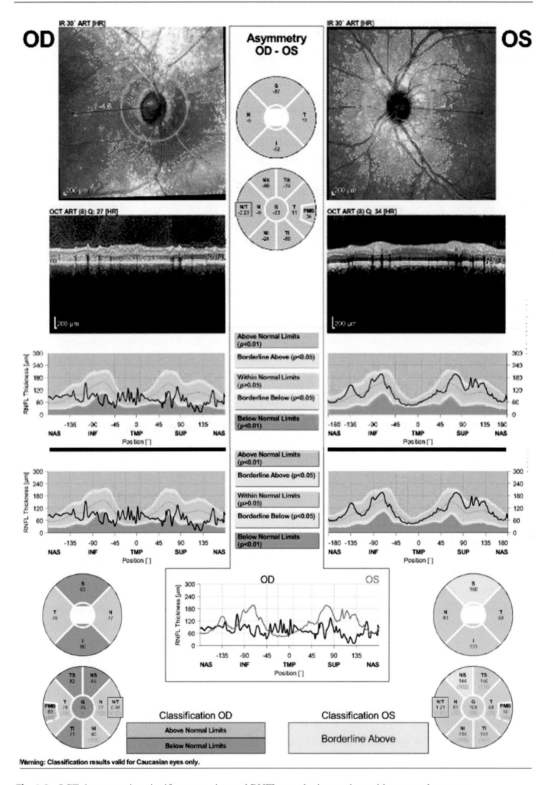

Fig. 1.2 OCT demonstrating significant cupping and RNFL atrophy in a patient with severe glaucoma

Multiple Sclerosis

Episodes of optic neuritis often show up on OCT as optic disk edema. As optic neuritis resolves and turns into optic pallor, this can also be seen on OCT as a relative loss of the nerve fiber layer.

OCT can be helpful in patients with remitting relapsing multiple sclerosis to detect new bouts of optic neuritis. This quantitative measure of optic nerve swelling can be especially useful in patients with concurrent ocular disorders that can contribute to decreased vision (Figs. 1.4 and 1.5).

Common Artifacts and Errors

1. Centering of the optic nerve around the scanner image

    RNFL thickness depends upon centering of the optic nerve, in order to achieve an accurate assessment of RNFL thickness. Lack of centering contributes to inaccurate overall RNFL measurements. Typically, the RNFL becomes falsely thicker in the quadrant in which the scan is closer to the disk and thinner in the quadrant in which the scan is displaced further from the disk [17]. Additionally, improper centering makes the reproducibility of scans more variable.

2. RNFL thickness in hypoplastic optic disks, enlarged optic disks, and myopic optic disks

    RNFL algorithms also depend on the presence of a relatively "normal" sized optic disk. With smaller optic disks, the RNFL thickness measurement typically declines and can create the appearance of thinner overall RNFL measurements. With larger optic disks, the RNFL thickness measurements increase, perhaps due to shorter distance between the circular scan and the optic disk edge [18]. With myopic disks, RNFL thickness can also be thinner and variable, resulting in a higher amount of false positives with routine glaucoma screening [19]. This important concept should be kept in mind when interpreting any OCT scan.

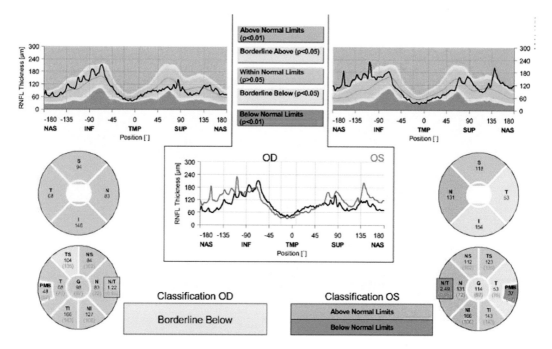

Fig. 1.3 Retinal nerve fiber layer measurements in a patient with idiopathic intracranial hypertension, showing presence of increased edema in the left optic nerve as compared to the right optic nerve

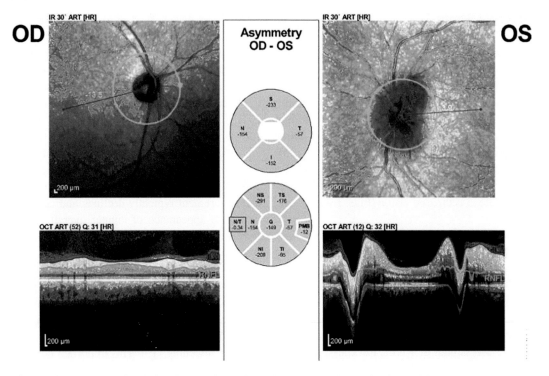

Fig. 1.4 Severe edema of the left optic nerve in a patient with an acute episode of optic neuritis

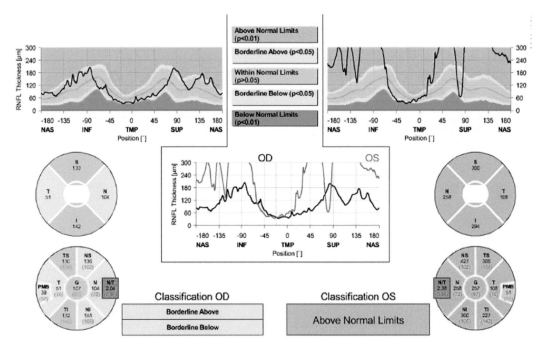

Fig. 1.5 Retinal nerve fiber layer measurements in a patient with an acute episode of optic neuritis in the left eye, reflecting the presence of severe edema in the left optic nerve

3. Algorithm error

RNFL thickness is based on an algorithm that calculates the anterior border of the RNFL. However, occasionally, this algorithm can pick up incorrect or inaccurate RNFL parameters, whether due to marked RNFL edema that distorts the underlying retina and choroid, or due to vitreous overlying the RNFL. A tip-off to an algorithm error is when the RNFL graph goes out of range (red arrow) or to zero baseline (blue arrow) (Fig. 1.6).

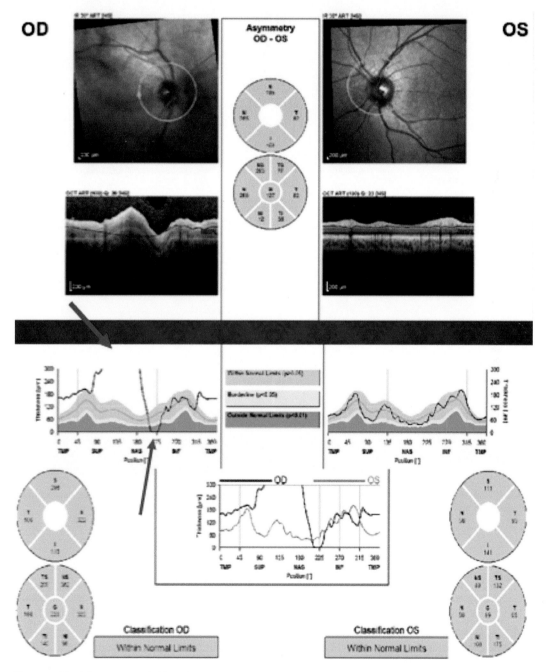

Fig. 1.6 Algorithm error on OCT. A tip-off to an algorithm error is when the RNFL graph goes out of range (*red arrow*) or to zero baseline (*blue arrow*)

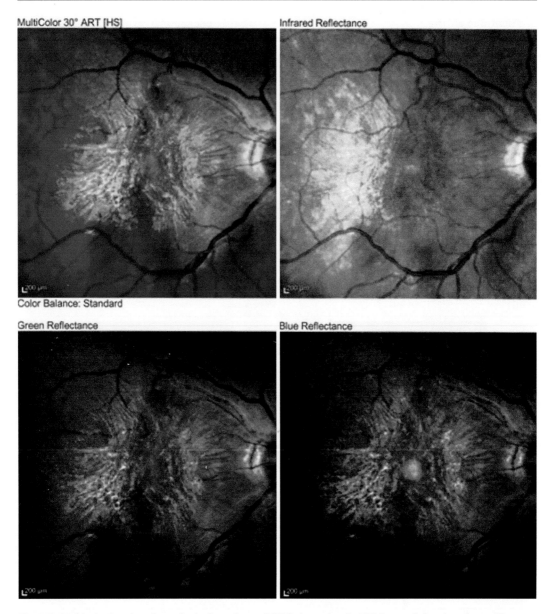

Fig. 1.7 Multicolor imaging of an epiretinal membrane (ERM) shows that the ERM not only involves the papillomacular bundle but also most of the macula. Differing depths can be appreciated by using multicolor imaging

4. RNFL measurements that exceed the software of the OCT device

   Rarely, as a disease process progresses, it outgrows the ability to detect change on OCT. This typically happens at very low measurements (extreme atrophy of RNFL) or very high measurements (extreme edema and swelling of the RNFL). At these very high or very low measurements, there is less validity of changes in the RNFL.

5. Maculopathies and neuropathies affecting macular thickness scans and nerve fiber layer measurements

   An important point to keep in mind is that a maculopathy that affects the retina and causes an overall decrease in the nerve fiber layer and ganglion cell layer will also decrease RNFL measurements at the optic nerve. Similarly, a condition which causes atrophy of RNFL at the optic nerve will also cause a thinning of the outer retinal layers throughout the macula.

Introduction to Multicolor OCT

Multicolor OCT is increasingly gaining interest among ophthalmologists. Confocal scanning laser ophthalmoscopy is utilized at three different wavelengths: blue (486 nm), green (518 nm), and infrared (IR; 815 nm) to reconstruct a series of images of varying retinal depth [4]. The different colored wavelengths penetrate at different levels to create detailed images of retinal layers. The blue light provides detailed images of superficial retina, including the retinal nerve fiber layer, ganglion cell layer, and epiretinal membranes. The green light penetrates deeper and is strongly absorbed by hemoglobin and therefore provides detailed images of midretinal layers, blood vessels, hemorrhage, and exudates. Finally, red light provides the most depth of penetration and provides images of the choroid, retinal pigment epithelium, and photoreceptors (Fig. 1.7).

Disclosure Dr. Sergott is a paid consultant to Heidelberg Engineering as well as the recipient of research funding. He has participated in the development process of several optic nerve and retinal imaging technologies. He does not hold any patents and receives no royalties from Heidelberg Engineering.

References

1. Huang D, Swanson EA, Lin CP, Schuman JS, Stinson WG, Chang W, et al. Optical coherence tomography. Science. 1991;254(5036):1178–81.
2. Fujimoto JG, Pitris C, Boppart SA, Brezinkski ME. Optical coherence tomography: an emerging technology for biomedical imaging and optical biopsy. Neoplasia. 2000;2(1–2):9–25.
3. Ishibazawa A, Nagaoka T, Takahashi A, Omae T, Tani T, Sogawa K, et al. Optical coherence tomography angiography in diabetic retinopathy: a prospective pilot study. Am J Ophthalmol. 2015;160(1):35–44.
4. Moussa NB, Georges A, Capuano V, Merle B, Souied EH, Querques G. Multicolor imaging in the evaluation of geographic atrophy due to age-related macular degeneration. Br J Ophthalmol. 2015;99(6):842–7.
5. Staurenghi G, Sadda S, Chakravarthy U, Spaide RF, International Nomenclature for Optical Coherence Tomography Panel. Proposed lexicon for anatomic landmarks in normal posterior segment spectral-domain optical coherence tomography. The IN OCT Consensus. Ophthalmology. 2014;121(8):1572–8.
6. Tibbets MD, Reichel E, Witkin AJ. Vision loss after intravitreal ocriplasmin: correlation of spectral-domain optical coherence tomography and electroretinography. JAMA Ophthalmol. 2014;132(4):487–90.
7. Sharma P, Juhn A, Houston SK, Fineman M, Chiang A, Ho A, et al. Efficacy of ocriplasmin for vitreomacular traction and full-thickness macular hole. Am J Ophthalmol. 2015;159(5):861–7.
8. Kerrison JB. Optic neuropathies caused by toxins and adverse drug reactions. Ophthalmol Clin North Am. 2004;17:481–8.
9. Vieira LM, Silva NF, Dias Dos Santos AM, Anjos RS, Abegao Pinto LA, Vincente AR, et al. Retinal ganglion cell layer analysis by optical coherence tomography in toxic and nutritional optic neuropathy. J Neuroophthalmol. 2015;3:242–5.
10. Marmor MF, Kellner U, Lai TYY, Lyons JS, Mieler WF, American Academy of Ophthalmology. Revised recommendations on screening for chloroquine and hydroxychloroquine retinopathy. Ophthalmology. 2011;118:415–22.
11. Chen E, Brown DM, Benz MS, Fish RH, Wong TP, Kim RY, et al. Spectral domain optical coherence tomography as an effective screening test for hydroxychloroquine retinopathy (the "flying saucer" sign). Clin Ophthalmol. 2010;4:1151–8.
12. Sarac O, Tasci YY, Gurdal C, Can I. Differentiation of optic disc edema from optic nerve head drusen with spectral-domain optical coherence tomography. J Neuroophthalmol. 2012;32(3):207–11.
13. Silverman AL, Tatham AJ, Medeiros FA, Weinreb RN. Assessment of optic nerve head drusen using enhanced depth imaging and swept source optical coherence tomography. J Neuroophthalmol. 2014; 34(2):198–205.
14. Wu Z, Xu G, Weinreb RN, Yu M, Leung CK. Optic nerve head deformation in glaucoma: a prospective analysis of optic nerve head surface and lamina cribrosa surface displacement. Ophthalmology. 2015;122(7):1317–29.
15. Bussel II, Wollstein G, Schuman JS. OCT for glaucoma diagnosis, screening and detection of glaucoma progression. Br J Ophthalmol. 2014;98 Suppl 2:ii15–9.
16. Kaufhold F, Kadas EM, Schmidt C, Kunte H, Hoffmann J, Zimmermann H, et al. Optic nerve head quantification in idiopathic intracranial hypertension by spectral domain OCT. PLoS One. 2012; 7(5):e36965.

17. Vizzeri G, Bowd C, Medeiros FA, Weinreb RN, Zangwill LM. Effect of improper scan alignment on retinal nerve fiber layer measurements using Stratus optical coherence tomograph. J Glaucoma. 2008;17(5):341–9.

18. Savini G, Zanini M, Carelli V, Sadun AA, Ross-Cisneros FN, Barboni P. Correlation between retinal nerve fibre layer thickness and optic nerve head size: an optical coherence tomography study. Br J Ophthalmol. 2005;89(4):489–92.

19. Vernon SA, Rotchford AP, Negi A, Ryatt S, Tattersal C. Peripapillary retinal nerve fibre layer thickness in highly myopic caucasians as measured by Stratus optical coherence tomography. Br J Ophthalmol. 2008;92(8):1076–80.

Macular Degeneration

Daniel W. Upton

Abstract

Age-related macular degeneration (ARMD) is the leading cause of loss of central visual acuity in those greater than 60 years old. In 2004, the prevalence was estimated at 1.6 million US citizens by Friedman (2011) and the number only continues to rise. Ocular coherence tomography (OCT) has been a major diagnostic tool in the identification and management of ARMD since its inception. As spectral domain OCT has replaced time-domain OCT, more in-depth imaging has continued to help redefine this disease. This entity has been invaluable since the emergence of anti-vascular endothelial growth factor (VEGF) therapy for exudative disease although now it has also shown a more significant role in nonexudative disease. Parafoveal telangiectasia (PFT) is a similar appearing entity to ARMD leading to the two occasionally being confused with one another especially when PFT leads to choroidal neovascular membrane. This entity was originally described by Gass in 1982 and was previously detected by clinical exam and fluorescence angiography, but with spectral domain OCT (SD-OCT) it is more easily recognizable with less invasive testing. It shows OCT triad of thinning, loss of the IS/OS junction, and cystoids. Overall, SD-OCT has revolutionized the detection and the evaluation of progression/regression of ARMD and parafoveal telangiectasia.

Keywords

Macular degeneration • Juxtafoveal telangiectasia • Parafoveal telangiectasia

D.W. Upton, MD
Department of Ophthalmology,
Geisinger Medical Center, Danville, PA, USA
e-mail: dwupton@geisinger.edu

© Springer International Publishing Switzerland 2016
A. Girach, R.C. Sergott (eds.), *Optical Coherence Tomography*,
DOI 10.1007/978-3-319-24817-2_2

Age-Related Macular Degeneration

Age-related macular degeneration (ARMD) is the leading cause of loss of central visual acuity in those greater than 60 years old. In 2004, the prevalence was estimated at 1.6 million US citizens by Friedman et al. [1] and the number only continues to rise. Ocular coherence tomography (OCT) has been a major diagnostic tool in the identification and management of ARMD since its inception. As spectral domain OCT (SD-OCT) has replaced time-domain OCT, more in-depth imaging has continued to help redefine this disease. This entity has been invaluable since the emergence of antivascular endothelial growth factor (VEGF) therapy for exudative disease although now it has also shown a more significant role in nonexudative disease.

Nonexudative ARMD OCT

The hallmark of this disease is drusen, which are deposits of extracellular material between Bruch's membrane and the retinal pigment epithelium (RPE) (Fig. 2.1). These were either unable to be seen or if seen unable to be well defined by time-domain OCT, but with SD-OCT, these can be seen and measured in both thickness and in area. The most common drusen (80 % per Yehohua et al. [2]) show characteristics of being convex, homogenous, having medium internal

reflectivity, and having no overlying hyperreflectivity. However, there can be many different combinations of drusen characteristics seen on imaging. The retina overlying the drusen shows photoreceptor thinning per Schuman et al. [3], but it is uncertain as to whether this indicates retinal degeneration versus simple displacement and/or compression of the photoreceptors. 3D reconstructions now allow for the combination of global retinal view and specific line scans simultaneously (Figs. 2.2 and 2.3), therefore yielding further ability to extrapolate volumetric data of drusen. Fundus autofluorescence shows hyperfluorescence at drusen due to their high lipofuscin content and can also show atrophy well as hypoautofluorescence (Fig. 2.4).

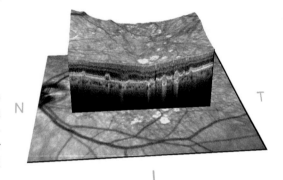

Fig. 2.2 Three-dimensional view and nonexudative ARMD showing a combination of drusen and atrophy with overlying retinal surface view showing the other areas of disease throughout the fundus. *N* nasal, *T* Temporal, *I* Inferior

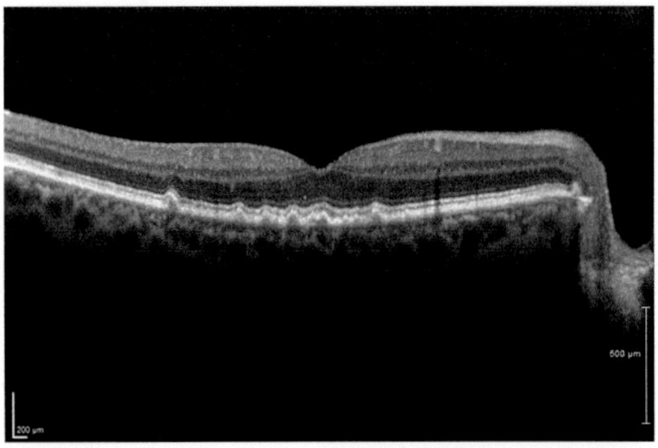

Fig. 2.1 A typical nonexudative ARMD with multiple drusen throughout the perifoveal area showing undulations in the IS/OS junction and the external limiting membrane. But has little to no effect on internal retinal structures

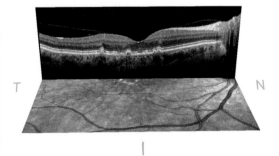

Fig. 2.3 Nonexudative ARMD with many drusen shown as a 3D view of an individual line scan so that one can see the multiple drusen present in the line scan but also other drusen seen in the macula via the retinal surface projection. *N* nasal, *T* Temporal, *I* Inferior

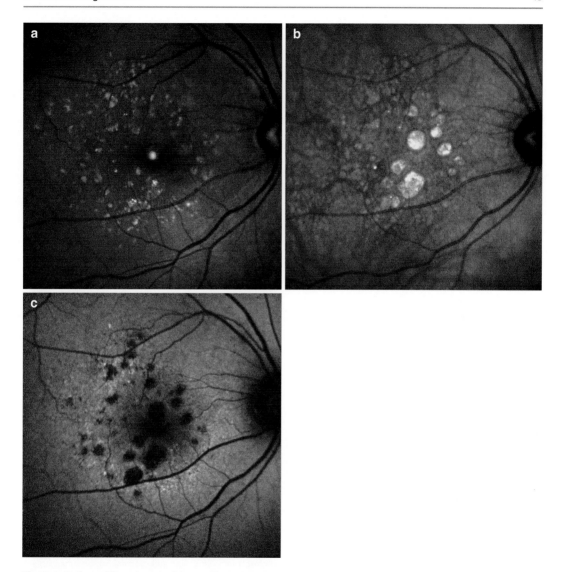

Fig. 2.4 Patient with nongeographic atrophy with areas of drusen intermixed with small areas of atrophy with RPE dropout comparing red-free (**a**), infrared (**b**), and fundus autofluorescence (**c**)

Geographic Atrophy Nonexudative ARMD OCT

SD-OCT can assess geographic atrophy best by looking at the 3D cube giving a summation of all the A and B scans. Geographic atrophy appears as bright areas in the macula based on loss of the RPE and choriocapillaris, which typically scatter light, therefore allowing transmission to the choroid. The increased transmission to the choroid appears as brighter, more defined choroidal architecture as well as deeper penetration than the surrounding

normal tissue (Fig. 2.5). This area can also be examined by cycling through the individual raster line scans assessing for loss of RPE with overlying photoreceptor degeneration seen by loss of the inner segment/outer segment line (Fig. 2.6).

Geographic Atrophy Fundus Autofluorescence

Fundus autofluorescence has emerged as an excellent way to assess nonexudative disease that

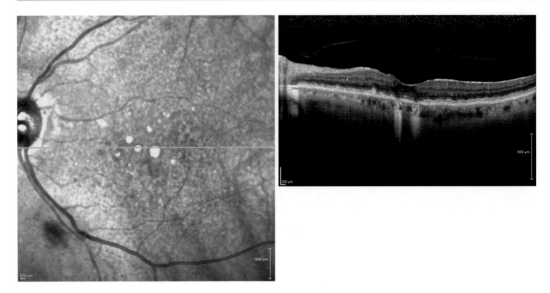

Fig. 2.5 Nonexudative ARMD showing multiple drusen as well as RPE dropout centrally leading to light transmission and significantly more choroidal signal at the edges of the fovea in areas of dropout

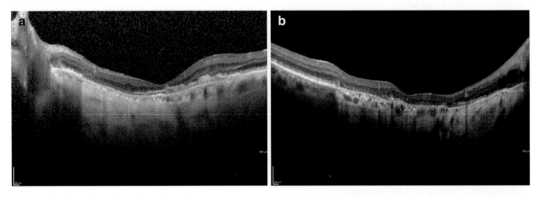

Fig. 2.6 Geographic atrophy line scan of patient's left (**a**) and right (**b**) eye showing irregular thin retina with loss of RPE allowing significant signal penetration well into the choroid. The transition from normal to atrophic retina is readily identifiable by the abrupt loss of posterior retinal architecture (IS/OS line and external limiting membrane) and increased choroidal signal

takes on a geographic atrophy pattern. Geographic atrophy appears as hypoautofluorescent areas due to loss of lipofuscin (the most common fluorophore in the posterior pole) (Fig. 2.7). Interestingly, this hypoautofluorescence often extends further then that seen on exam (Figs. 2.8 and 2.9). Autofluorescence also shows extent of disease more clearly than other modalities (Figs. 2.10 and 2.11). Some drawbacks include difficulty to detect with moderate cataracts (although this is improving with newer machines), difficulty with identifying in the foveal/parafoveal region due to retinal xanthophylls located there that normally block FAF, and the assumption that hypoautofluorescence identically mirrors RPE dysfunction.

Exudative Disease

Neovascular age-related macular degeneration is the minority of ARMD comprising 15–20 % of the disease but has a disproportionate amount of the severe vision loss. This entity is where OCT has

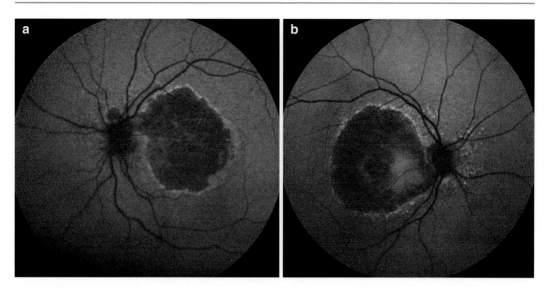

Fig. 2.7 Fundus autofluorescence of bilateral geographic atrophy (**a**, right eye; **b**, left eye) with large area of lost RPE leading to hypofluorescence with sickened RPE along the edge of atrophic area seen as hyperfluorescence

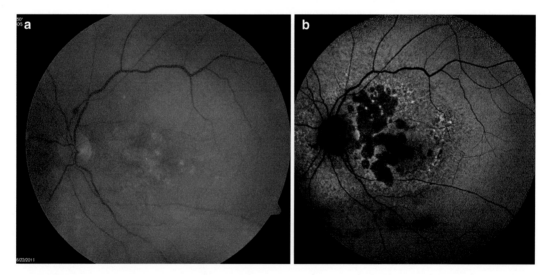

Fig. 2.8 Patient with significant macular atrophy seen both by fundus photography (**a**) and fundus autofluorescence (**b**). This exemplifies how FAF shows superiority in demonstrating extent of atrophic disease as nondescript boundaries on photo become clear on FAF

become an essential tool for diagnosis and treatment due to the emergence of anti-VEGF therapies. Classic CNV fibrovascular tissue presents as a defined hyperreflective area that is located between RPE and Bruch's membrane and/or extending through RPE into the subretinal space. Occult disease is more often an RPE elevation from serous fluid or fibrovascular tissue at the choroidal plane. This can be compared to a simple pigment epithelial detachment as seen in Fig. 2.12. In either circumstance, active disease is associated with adjacent fluid in the sub-RPE and subretinal spaces as well as associated retinal edema in any retinal layer (Figs. 2.13, 2.14, 2.15, 2.16, 2.17, 2.18, 2.19, 2.20, and 2.21). Types of neovascularization have been adjusted to incorporate the new findings that SD-OCT has shown. Type 1 includes CNV in the sub-RPE space most consistent with

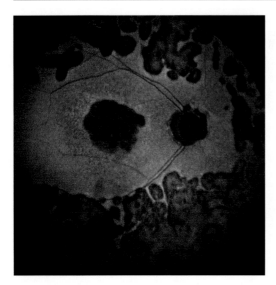

Fig. 2.9 Fundus autofluorescence demonstrating central geographic atrophy with extensive PRP-induced chorioretinal scarring also seen in this diabetic patient. You can see that the geographic atrophy (GA) is more hypofluorescent with loss of the RPE, whereas the scars show some hyperfluorescence from RPE hypertrophy intermixed with hypofluorescence from dropout

occult disease, type 2 characterized by CNV in the subretinal space most consistent with classic disease, and finally, type 3 is characterized by intraretinal neovascularization. All of the forms of exudative disease tend to respond well to anti-VEGF therapy although pigment epithelial detachments tend to be more difficult to treat (Figs. 2.22 and 2.23). One possible complication of therapy especially in the case of fibrovascular PED is an RPE tear where the RPE scrolls up creating elevation and leaves adjacent atrophy where the RPE has scrolled from (Figs. 2.24 and 2.25). The elevated RPE shows significant blocking of light and choroid is not seen posterior to this. In cases of RPE, tears typically see rapid and significant decline in central vision.

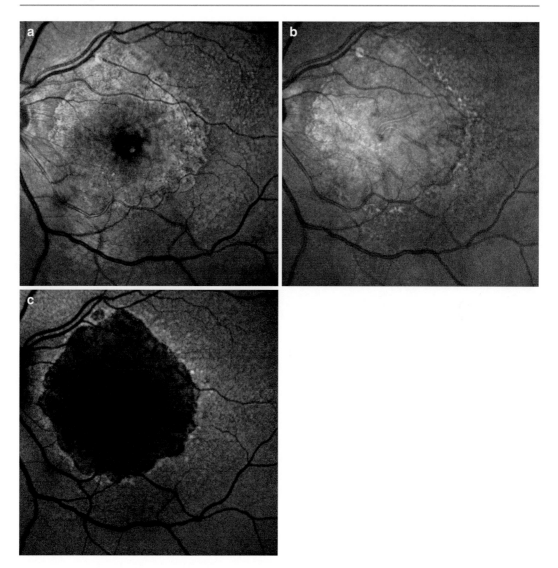

Fig. 2.10 Red-free (**a**), infrared (**b**), and fundus autofluorescence (**c**) of geographic atrophy demonstrating increasing ease of determining extent of with fundus autofluorescence showing superiority versus other two modalities

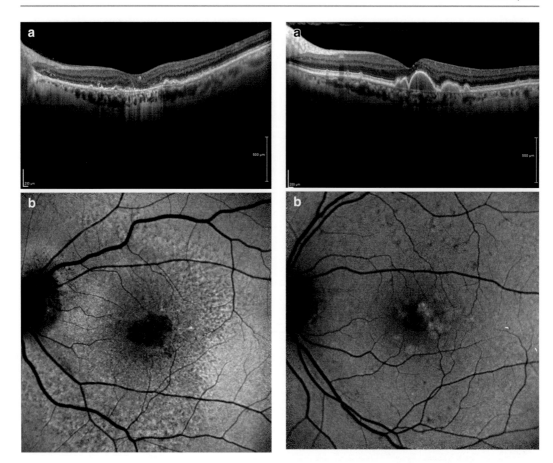

Fig. 2.11 Central geographic atrophy seen as loss of outer retinal architecture with increased choroidal penetration on raster line scan (**a**) corresponding to hypoautofluorescence on FAF (**b**). Also demonstrated on the autofluorescence is multiple drusen seen as small hyperfluorescent spots

Fig. 2.12 ARMD showing several large pigment epithelial detachments (PED) without any adjacent subretinal or intraretinal edema demonstrated well on line scan (**a**) and seen as areas of hyperautofluorescence in the FAF (**b**)

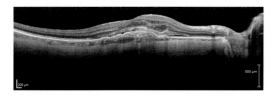

Fig. 2.13 Classic exudative ARMD showing large hyperreflective sub-RPE membrane with subretinal fluid and small area of intraretinal edema nasal to the fovea within the inner nuclear layer

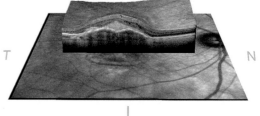

Fig. 2.14 3D view of exudative ARMD demonstrating CNV with retinal thickening and edema on line scan but also demonstrating area of involvement with superimposed retinal surface image. *N* nasal, *T* Temporal, *I* Inferior

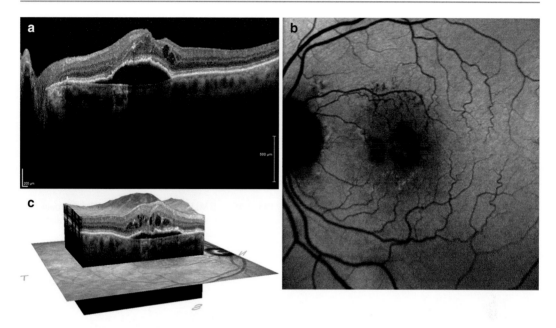

Fig. 2.15 Exudative disease seen in both line scan (**a**) showing large PED with associated intraretinal edema and by fundus autofluorescence (**b**) showing increased fluorescence centrally as well as underlying drusen and atrophy. The 3D rendering (**c**) demonstrates topographic changes, extent of disease, as well as edema and subretinal fluid. *N* nasal, *T* Temporal, *I* Inferior

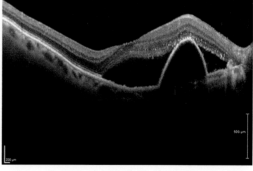

Fig. 2.17 Peripapillary choroidal neovascular membrane seen as large serous pigment epithelial detachment in the perifoveal region with significant subretinal fluid extending under the fovea. Differential for this should also include polypoidal choroidopathy and central serous chorioretinopathy

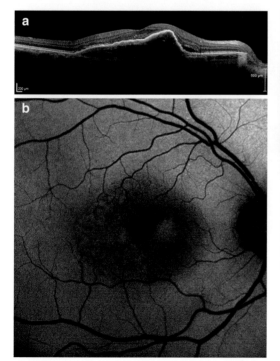

Fig. 2.16 Massive subfoveal choroidal neovascular membrane creating fibrovascular PED and subretinal fluid. Line scan (**a**) shows vertical extent of PED, adjacent subretinal fluid, and retinal distortion. Fundus autofluorescence (**b**) shows fluid as increased autofluorescence on FAF in the perifoveal region

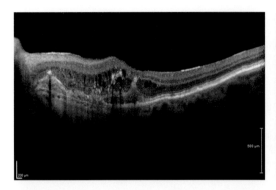

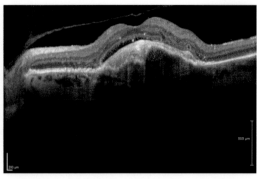

Fig. 2.18 Severe exudative ARMD with CNV in the nasal macula extending into the foveal region with loss of outer retinal architecture and significant outer nuclear layer edema

Fig. 2.19 ARMD with large fibrovascular pigment epithelial detachment with adjacent subretinal fluid and some mild intraretinal fluid temporally

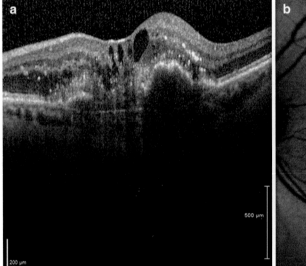

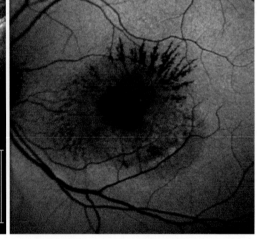

Fig. 2.20 Large choroidal neovascular membrane with significant retinal edema. Retinal hemorrhage seen as hyperfluorescent areas on the line scan (**a**). Fundus auto-fluorescence (**b**) shows bleeding that appears hypofluorescent radiating from perifoveal area and some scattered increased autofluorescence in the perifoveal area

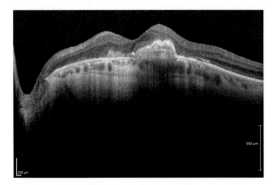

Fig. 2.21 End-stage exudative ARMD leaving hyperreflective scar within the outer retina without adjacent edema or subretinal fluid in area of previous exudation

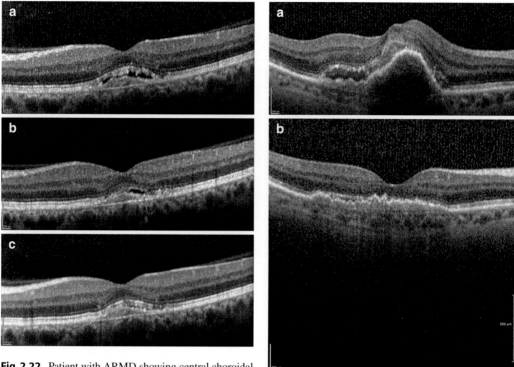

Fig. 2.22 Patient with ARMD showing central choroidal neovascular membrane with adjacent subretinal fluid seen initially (**a**) at 2 weeks (**b**) and at 2 months (**c**) after getting monthly Avastin injections. Subretinal fluid partially resolved at 2 weeks and almost completely resolved at 2 months which corresponded to much improvement in vision clinically

Fig. 2.23 Patient showing severe exudative ARMD when initially seen (**a**). Large PED with adjacent fibrovascular consistency to the subretinal space. Posttreatment (**b**) shows that the PED has greatly improved with only the small fibrovascular area in the subretinal space remaining

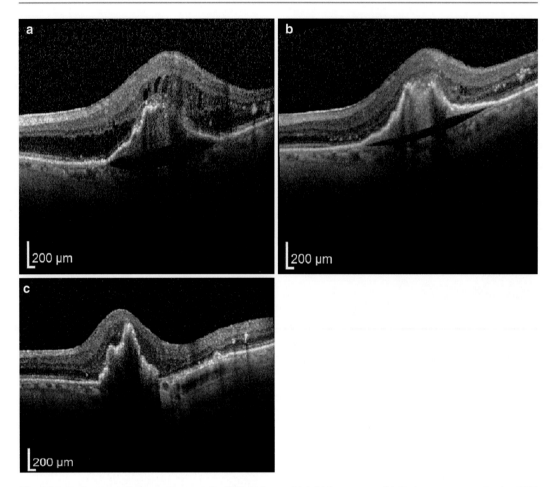

Fig. 2.24 Patient seen for large fibrovascular PED indicating CNV in the sub-RPE space with large subretinal fluid collection and retinal edema (**a**). Edema resolves with initial treatments (**b**). Patient went on to develop RPE tear with bunched-up RPE leading to significant elevation and adjacent RPE loss (**c**)

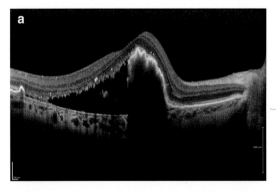
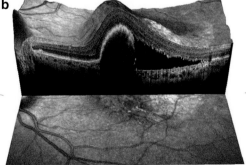

Fig. 2.25 Patient with long-standing exudative macular degeneration now post multiple anti-VEGF injections presents with large RPE tear. This is shown as a raster line scan (**a**) and a three-dimensional reconstruction (**b**). RPE scrolled nasally leading to a large ridge of RPE tissue elevating the retina and completely blocking the view of the choroid below. Atrophy is seen temporal to the elevation where RPE has been pulled into the scrolled segment leaving no pigment epithelium and degenerated photoreceptors

Parafoveal Telangiectasia

History

Parafoveal telangiectasia is a condition that leads to retinal degeneration and disorganization in the perifoveal region resulting in decreased visual acuity and/or metamorphopsia. It was first recognized by Gass and Oyakawa in 1982 [4]. It was originally described as bilateral paracentral capillary telangiectasia of unknown cause by Gass. Although further knowledge has been gained over the past 31 years, the exact etiology of this condition remains elusive. Gass proposed three groups with subclasses within. Group 1 consists of a congenital disease with male predominance (10:1) that is typically unilateral with greater than 2 disk diameters of telangiectasias with some degree of associated edema and exudate. Typically, this has little effect on best-corrected visual acuity (BCVA). Many feel that this is a subset of Coats disease that acts more focally than the classic disease. Group 2 is the most common by far but is still rare with prevalence of 0.1 % [5]. It consists of bilateral symmetric capillary changes in an area less than one disk diameter just temporal to the fovea. It occasionally shows crystalline-like deposits similar to the iridescent Muller cell foot plates seen in retinoschisis. Finally, it can also show significant RPE changes and associated choroidal neovascular membrane. It has no gender predominance and typically shows an onset in fifth to seventh decade of life with BCVA in the 20/40-20/70 range. Group 3 is an extremely rare condition, with bilateral symmetric perifoveal obliterative vasculitis associated with entities such as polycythemia, gout, ulcerative colitis, multiple myeloma, and chronic lymphocytic leukemia. The disease was originally diagnosed on clinical exam demonstrating dilated capillary beds, RPE changes, and/or exudates. Fluorescein angiogram (FA) demonstrated these dilated capillary beds well with early hyperfluorescence and late leakage. The widespread institution of OCT was able to show retinal changes in this disease without the inva-siveness that is inherent in angiography. As the imaging revolution continued and spectral domain OCT emerged, more defined images captured the changes that occur in this disease and provoked further questions into the etiology and pathophysiology of this entity.

OCT Characteristics

The OCT characteristics vary by group. Discussion will begin with group 2 as this is by far the most common presentation. The typical appearance includes:

- Thinning of the photoreceptor layer or loss of the IS/OS line (Figs. 2.26 and 2.27)
- Cystoids (Figs. 2.26 and 2.27)
- Reduced foveal thickness (Fig. 2.28)

It is still not well understood what leads to these changes, but the leading theories converge on a final point of Mueller cell dysfunction subsequently leading to lose of the retinal tissue that these cells nourish. The cystoids appear as edema on OCT, but based on FA and histology findings

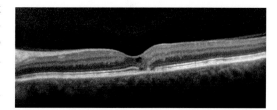

Fig. 2.26 Line scan through fovea of type 2 parafoveal telangiectasia showing loss of the IS/OS line temporal to the fovea with cystoid space above in the overlying inner retina with ILM draped overtop

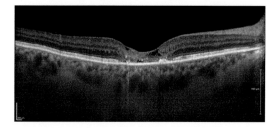

Fig. 2.27 Raster line scan through fovea of type 2 parafoveal telangiectasia showing significant foveal thinning, loss of the IS/OS line, and cystoids in the inner retina

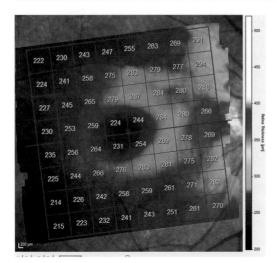

Fig. 2.28 Posterior pole thickness map showing significant thinning in the temporal parafoveal region, a classic finding in parafoveal telangiectasias

are actually areas of retinal loss with draping of the ILM/inner retinal layers overtop (Fig. 2.29).

Finally, RPE changes open a window for choroidal neovascularization and therefore can show

the appearance identical to that seen in ARMD with hemorrhage, subretinal fluid, and intraretinal fluid. This disease tends to lack pigment epithelial detachments (PED) (Fig. 2.30).

Group 1 is a less common form of this condition and is a Coats disease-like appearance in a contained area. On OCT, there is typically some degree of cystoid macular edema. Many times there can be a sensory retinal serous detachment focally in the perifoveal region. It can appear similar to central serous chorioretinopathy, diabetic macular edema, and exudative age-related macular degeneration.

Fundus autofluorescence findings can be seen extremely early before clinical or other OCT changes occur. Changes start with increased autofluorescence in the fovea and temporal to the fovea before any other findings (Fig. 2.31). This continues to become more prominent as the disease progresses. Once RPE changes begin to occur, autofluorescence takes on a more salt and pepper appearance with a spattering of decreased autofluorescence representing the RPE changes throughout the involved area (Fig. 2.31).

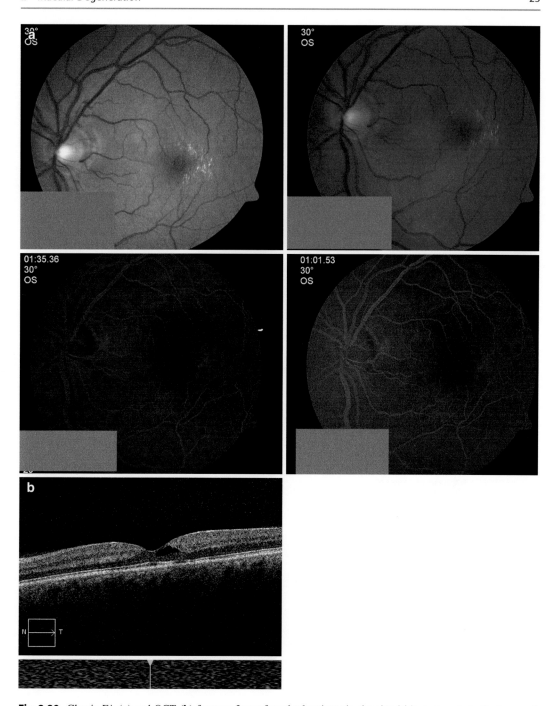

Fig. 2.29 Classic FA (**a**) and OCT (**b**) for type 2 parafoveal telangiectasia showing iridescent spots in the temporal perifoveal area with draping of the internal limiting membrane (ILM) over large cystoid space on OCT

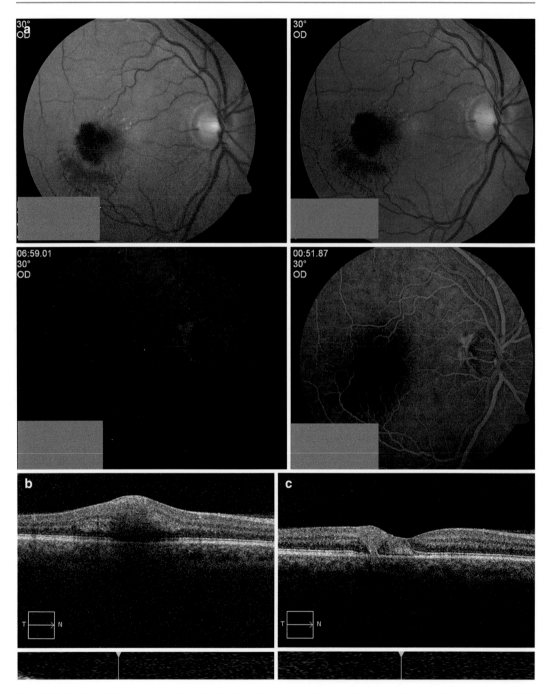

Fig. 2.30 Patient with type 2 parafoveal telangiectasia with associated CNV leading to retinal hemorrhage. FA (**a**) shows blocking by hemorrhage with late leakage at temporal edge of blocking. Initial OCT (**b**) with intraretinal hemorrhage and edema. One month post-Avastin OCT (**c**) showing resolution of the previous hemorrhage and edema now with loss of the IS/OS line consistent with underlying PFT

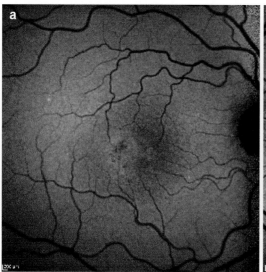

Fig. 2.31 Type 2 parafoveal telangiectasia bilateral fundus autofluorescence (*right* [**a**], *left* [**b**])showing mostly hyperfluorescence in the area of disease temporal to the fovea with some small hypofluorescent spots consistent with RPE changes

References

1. Friedman DS, O'Colmain BJ, Muñoz B, et al. Prevalence of age-related macular degeneration in the United States. Arch Ophthalmol. 2011;22:564–72.
2. Yehoshua Z, Rosenfeld PJ, Gregori G, Penha F. Spectral domain optical coherence tomography imaging of dry age-related macular degeneration. Ophthalmic Surg Lasers Imaging. 2010;41(Suppl):S6–14.
3. Schuman SG, Koreishi AF, Farsiu S, Jung SH, et al. Photoreceptor layer thinning over drusen in eyes with age related macular degeneration imaged in vivo with spectral domain optical coherence tomography. Ophthalmology. 2009;116:488–96.
4. Gass JD, Oyakawa RT. Idiopathic juxtafoveolar retinal telangiectasis. Arch Ophthalmol. 1982;100:769–80.
5. Klein R, Blodi BA, Meuer SM, Myers CE, et al. The prevalence of macular telangiectasia type 2 in the beaver dam eye study. Am J Ophthalmol. 2010;150:55–62.

Recommended Reading

Charbel Issa P, Finger RP, Kruse K, Baumüller S, Scholl HP, Holz FG. Monthly ranibizumab for nonproliferative macular telangiectasia type 2: a 12 month prospective study. Am J Ophthalmol. 2011;151:876–86.

Charbel Issa P, Gillies MC, Chew EY, Bird AC, Heeren TF, Peto T, Holz FG, Scholl HP. Macular telangiectasia type 2. Prog Retin Eye Res. 2013;34:49–77.
Gregori G, Wang F, Rosenfeld PJ, Yehoshua Z, et al. Spectral domain optical coherence tomography imaging of drusen in nonexudative age-related macular degeneration. Ophthalmology. 2011;118:1373–9.
Karadimas P, Bouzas EA. Fundus autofluorescence imaging in serous and drusenoid pigment epithelial detachments associated with age related macular degeneration. Am J Ophthalmol. 2005;140:1163–5.
Lois N, Owens SL, Coco R, Hopkins J, Fitzke FW, Bird AC. Fundus autofluorescence in patients with age related macular degeneration and high risk of visual loss. Am J Ophthalmol. 2002;133:341–9.
Nowilaty SR, Al-Shamsi HN, Al-Khars W. Idiopathic juxtafoveal retinal telangiectasis: a current review. Middle East Afr J Ophthalmol. 2010;17:224–41.
Regatieri CV, Branchini L, Duker JS. The role of spectral-domain OCT in the diagnosis and management of neovascular age-related macular degeneration. Ophthalmic Surg Lasers Imaging. 2011;42(Suppl):S56–66.
Schmitz-Valckenberg S, Fleckenstein M, Scholl HP, Holz FG. Fundus autofluorescence and progression of age related macular degeneration. Surv Ophthalmol. 2009;54:96–117.
Watzke RC, Klein ML, Folk JC, Farmer SG, Munsen RS, Champfer RJ, Sletten KR. Long-term juxtafoveal retinal telangiectasia. Retina. 2005;25:727–35.

Diabetic Retinopathy

M. Ali Khan and Alexander Juhn

Abstract

Diabetic retinopathy is the most common microvascular complication of diabetes mellitus. Of its varying manifestations, diabetic macular edema (DME) is the most frequent cause of vision loss in these patients. Optical coherence tomography (OCT) allows for the characterization and monitoring of DME, tractional retinal detachment, epiretinal membrane formation, and diabetic papillopathy and serves as an objective measure to which clinical decisions regarding treatment for these conditions can be determined. Illustrative cases will be presented.

Keywords

Diabetic macular edema • Tractional retinal detachment • Diabetic papillopathy

Introduction

Diabetic retinopathy remains the leading cause of new vision loss and legal blindness in working-aged patients in the United States and developed countries [1]. As the rates of obesity and diabetes are only predicted to rise, the burden of disease cannot be understated [2]. Of the varying manifestations of diabetic retinopathy, including cataract formation and proliferative changes, diabetic macular edema (DME) is the most frequent mechanism of vision loss in these patients [3].

Optical coherence tomography (OCT) has allowed for characterization and monitoring of

M.A. Khan, MD (✉) • A. Juhn, MD
Department of Ophthalmology, Wills Eye Hospital,
Philadelphia, PA, USA
e-mail: akhan@willseye.org; alexjuhn1@gmail.com

© Springer International Publishing Switzerland 2016
A. Girach, R.C. Sergott (eds.), *Optical Coherence Tomography*,
DOI 10.1007/978-3-319-24817-2_3

disease severity in diabetic retinopathy, including diabetic macular edema, tractional retinal detachment, epiretinal membrane formation, and diabetic papillopathy. OCT has been particularly important in the management of diabetic macular edema. In clinical studies investigating the efficacy of anti-vascular endothelial growth factor (VEGF) therapy for the treatment of DME, central macular thickness as determined by OCT is routinely used as a primary study outcome [4–12].

Indeed, OCT has become integral in clinical decision-making in patients with diabetic retinopathy. The following cases reflect OCT findings commonly encountered in this patient population.

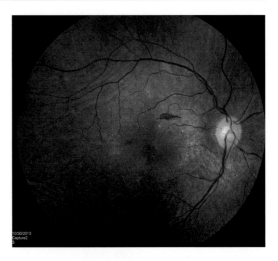

Fig. 3.1 Fundus photograph revealing clinically significant macular edema. Hard exudates, retinal thickening, and retinal hemorrhages are present

Diabetic Macular Edema

Diabetic macular edema (DME) is the result of abnormal retinal vascular permeability, evidenced histopathologically by loss of endothelial cells, loss of pericytes, and capillary basement membrane thickening [2]. DME may take many forms on OCT, manifesting in intraretinal, subretinal, and less frequently subretinal pigment epithelium fluid, with varying degrees of retinal structural alteration.

Case 1. Diabetic Macular Edema
Fundus examination of the right eye of an 81-year-old female with nonproliferative diabetic retinopathy reveals retinal thickening, intraretinal hemorrhages, and hard exudates consistent with macular edema (Fig. 3.1). The patient is pseudophakic, with a visual acuity of 20/30. Spectral domain OCT reveals both cystic intraretinal fluid and subretinal fluid, with alteration of the foveal contour (Fig. 3.2a–f).

Case 2. Diabetic Macular Edema
Fundus examination of the left eye of a 40-year-old female with nonproliferative diabetic retinopathy reveals impressive hard exudates and retinal thickening consistent with macular edema (Fig. 3.3). Hemoglobin A1c was noted to be 12.1 %, and visual acuity was 20/40. Spectral domain OCT reveals cystic intraretinal fluid

with hyperreflective spots correlating to retinal exudates (Fig. 3.4a–g) seen on fundoscopic exam. Macular thickness mapping illustrates the edema (Fig. 3.4h).

Case 3. Diabetic Macular Edema
Fundus examination of the right eye of a 51-year-old male with proliferative diabetic retinopathy reveals vitreous hemorrhage and numerous retinal hemorrhages and macular hard exudates (Fig. 3.5). Visual acuity was 20/200. Spectral domain OCT reveals impressive cystic intraretinal fluid. Outer retinal architecture is lost with attenuation of the ellipsoid layer (Fig. 3.6a–f).

Case 4. Diabetic Macular Edema
Spectral domain OCT (Fig. 3.7a–d) of the left eye of a 59-year-old male with nonproliferative diabetic retinopathy reveals small, central intraretinal cysts with hard exudates. Visual acuity was 20/20, and the patient was asymptomatic.

Case 5. Diabetic Macular Edema
A 47-year-old male was treated for diabetic macular edema (Fig. 3.8a) with a combination of anti-vascular endothelial growth factor and corticosteroid therapy. The edema improved, but loss of the ellipsoid layer was evident (Fig. 3.8b).

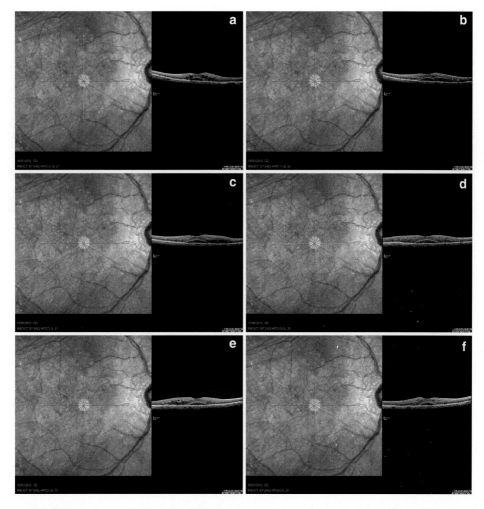

Fig. 3.2 (a–f) Spectral domain OCT axial images reveal intraretinal and subretinal fluid along with hyperreflective hard exudates

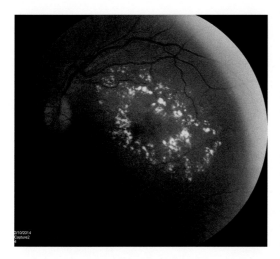

Fig. 3.3 Fundus photograph revealing impressive hard exudates and macular edema in a patient with non-proliferative diabetic retinopathy

Tractional Retinal Detachment

Tractional retinal detachment (TRD) is an advanced complication of proliferative diabetic retinopathy. OCT may be used to assess the extent of TRD and assess macular involvement.

Case 6. Tractional Retinal Detachment

Fundus examination of a 270-year-old female with proliferative diabetic retinopathy reveals chronic tractional retinal detachment in the left eye (Fig. 3.9). Spectral domain OCT demonstrates a shallow tractional retinal detachment (Fig. 3.10a–c). Fundus examination of the right eye in this same patient reveals a fibrovascular, tractional membrane overlying the optic nerve (Fig. 3.11). Spectral domain OCT demonstrates

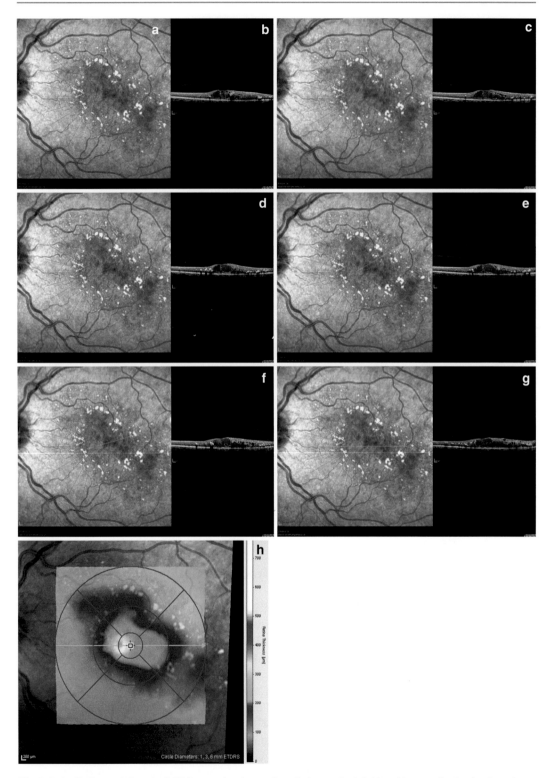

Fig. 3.4 (**a–h**) Spectral domain OCT images (**a–g**) reveal cystic intraretinal fluid and hyperreflective hard exudates. Macular mapping (**h**) illustrates well the associated retinal thickening

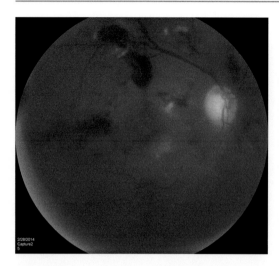

Fig. 3.5 Fundus photograph revealing proliferative diabetic retinopathy with vitreous hemorrhage and prominent retinal hemorrhages and hard exudates

this tractional band (Fig. 3.12). Visual acuity was hand motions in both eyes.

Case 7. Tractional Retinal Detachment
Enhanced depth imaging (EDI) spectral domain OCT reveals development of tractional retinal detachment (Fig. 3.13a–c). A 42-year-old male developed proliferative diabetic retinopathy and was noncompliant with follow-up and treatment recommendations. Imaging reveals subhyaloid hemorrhage and ultimately tractional retinal detachment. Near-infrared images highlight vascular proliferation.

Epiretinal Membrane

Case 8. Diabetic Macular Edema and Epiretinal Membrane
Fundus examination (Fig. 3.14) of the left eye of a 49-year-old male with proliferative diabetic retinopathy reveals hard exudates and retinal thickening consistent with macular edema. Spectral domain OCT reveals the presence of a concurrent epiretinal membrane (Fig. 3.15a–b). Visual acuity was 20/200.

Case 9. Diabetic Macular Edema and Epiretinal Membrane
Fundus examination (Fig. 3.16) of a 60-year-old male with proliferative diabetic retinopathy reveals retinal hemorrhages, hard exudates, sclerotic vessels, and an epiretinal membrane in the right eye. Spectral domain OCT reveals concurrent epiretinal membrane and diabetic macular edema (Fig. 3.17a–f). Hyperreflective hard exudates are also seen.

Diabetic Papillopathy

Diabetic papillopathy is characterized by unilateral or bilateral optic disk edema in patients with diabetes mellitus [13]. A diagnosis of exclusion, the precise pathophysiology remains uncertain, but this clinical entity has been characterized as an ischemic optic neuropathy [14]. Treatment using intravitreal corticosteroids and anti-vascular endothelial growth factor therapy has been described [15–17]. In similar fashion to DME, evaluation of the retinal nerve fiber layer thickness is useful for the quantification and monitoring of diabetic papillopathy.

Case 10. Diabetic Papillopathy
A 75-year-old female presented for evaluation of vision loss in the left eye progressing over 3 days. Medical history was significant only for non-insulin-dependent diabetes mellitus (hemoglobin A1c 10.1 %). Fundus examination revealed optic disk and macular edema in the left eye. Visual acuity was counting fingers and a relative afferent pupillary defect was present. Workup for other causes of optic disk edema with laboratory testing and MRI imaging was negative, and the diagnosis of diabetic papillopathy was made.

Spectral domain OCT reveals significant edema of the optic nerve head (Fig. 3.18a, b) with concurrent subretinal and intraretinal fluid in the macula (Fig. 3.19).

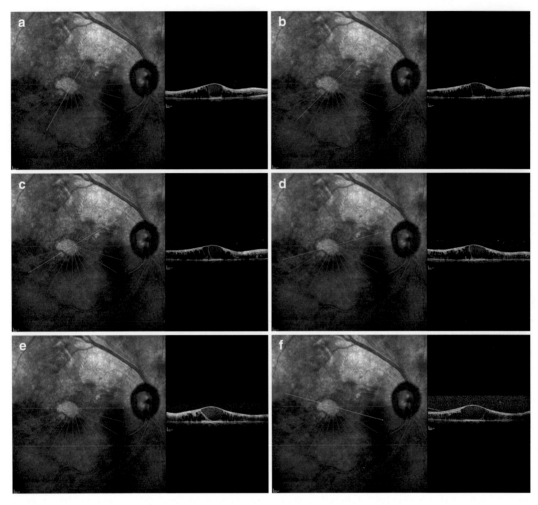

Fig. 3.6 (**a–f**) Spectral domain OCT images reveal impressive cystic intraretinal fluid with notable alteration of retinal architecture

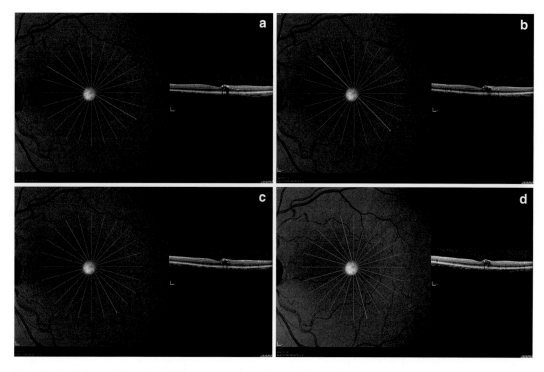

Fig. 3.7 (**a–d**) Spectral domain OCT images reveal small, central intraretinal cysts and associated hard exudates. The retinal architecture is largely preserved

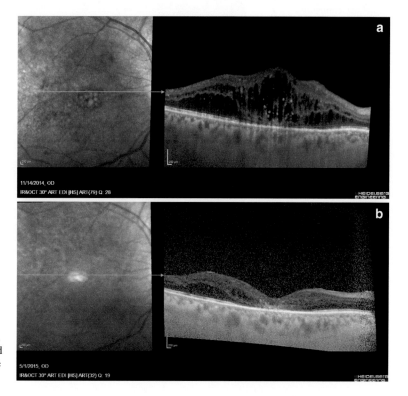

Fig. 3.8 (**a, b**) Spectral domain OCT reveals severe intraretinal cystic edema and loss of inner and outer retinal architecture. Edema improved with treatment, but loss of the ellipsoid layer was evident

Fig. 3.9 Fundus
photograph revealing
proliferative diabetic
retinopathy with tractional
retinal detachment. Prior
pan-retinal
photocoagulation is noted

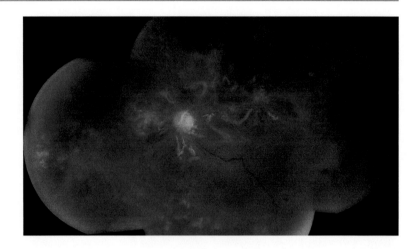

Fig. 3.10 (**a–c**) Spectral
domain OCT highlights a
tractional band and underlying
retinal detachment

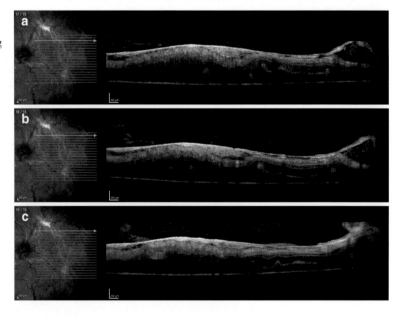

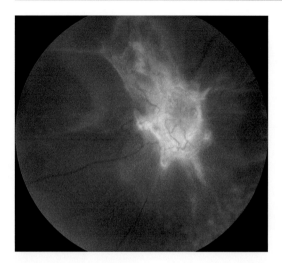

Fig. 3.11 Fundus photograph revealing a fibrovascular membrane overlying the optic nerve in a patient with proliferative diabetic retinopathy

Fig. 3.12 Spectral domain OCT illustrates a proliferative, fibrovascular membrane overlying the optic nerve

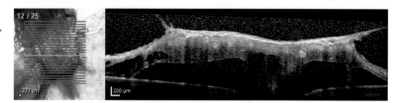

Fig. 3.13 (a–c) Spectral domain OCT reveals development of subhyaloid hemorrhage and subsequent tractional retinal detachment. Corresponding near-infrared images highlight development of vascular proliferation

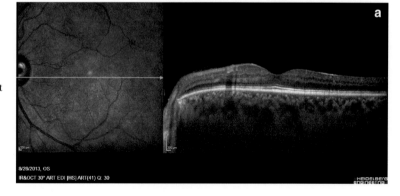

Fig. 3.13 (continued)

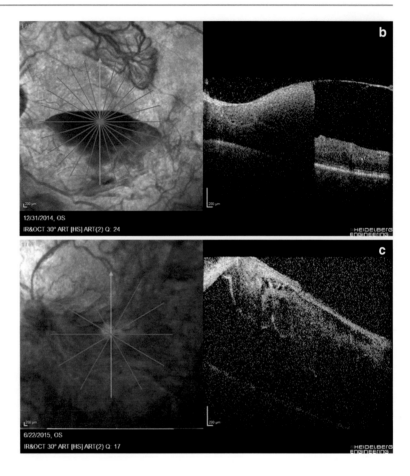

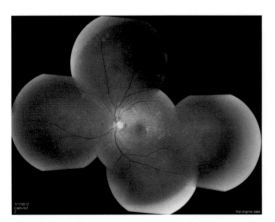

Fig. 3.14 Fundus photograph revealing non-proliferative diabetic retinopathy with clinically significant macular edema

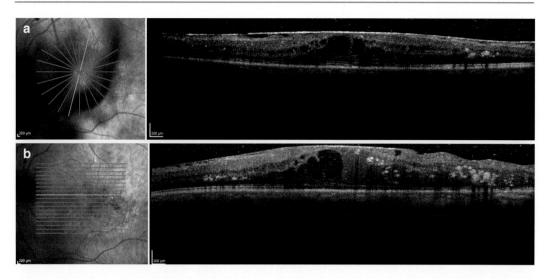

Fig. 3.15 (**a–b**) Spectral domain OCT highlights an epiretinal membrane with underlying cystic intraretinal fluid and hyperreflective hard exudates

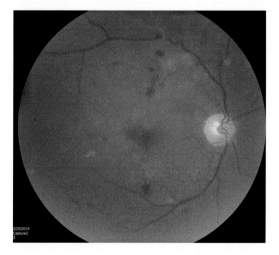

Fig. 3.16 Fundus photography reveals a macular epiretinal membrane along with retinal hemorrhages and hard exudates

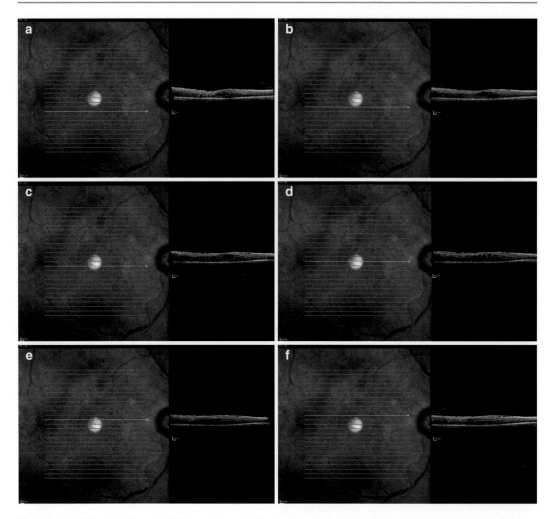

Fig. 3.17 (**a–f**) Spectral domain OCT reveals an epiretinal membrane with alteration of the foveal contour and under-lying cystic intraretinal fluid

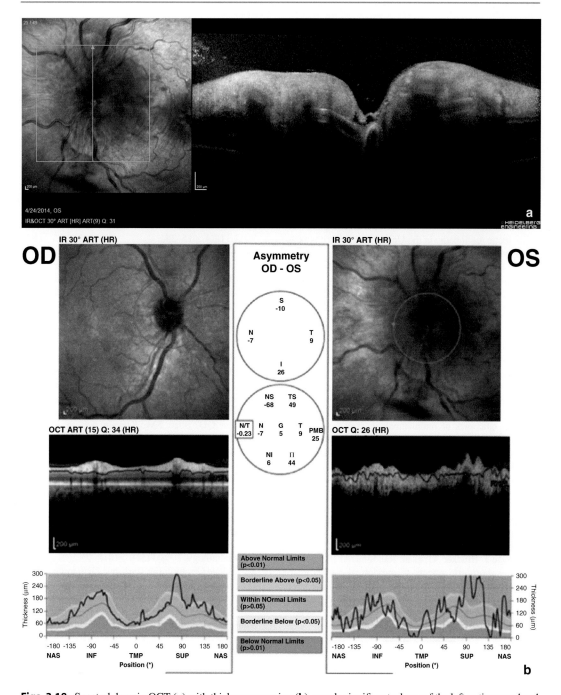

Fig. 3.18 Spectral domain OCT (**a**) with thickness mapping (**b**) reveals significant edema of the left optic nerve head

Fig. 3.19 Spectral domain OCT revealing edema of the optic nerve head and macula, with cystic intraretinal and subretinal fluid

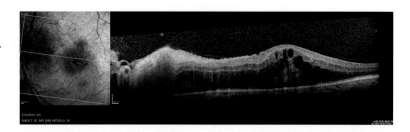

References

1. Zhang X, Saaddine JB, Chou C-F, et al. Prevalence of diabetic retinopathy in the United States, 2005–2008. JAMA. 2010;304(6):649–56.
2. Ho AC, Scott IU, Kim SJ, et al. Anti-vascular endothelial growth factor pharmacotherapy for diabetic macular edema: a report by the American Academy of Ophthalmology. Ophthalmology. 2012;119(10):2179–88.
3. Klein R, Klein BE, Moss SE, Cruickshanks KJ. The Wisconsin Epidemiologic Study of Diabetic Retinopathy: XVII. The 14-year incidence and progression of diabetic retinopathy and associated risk factors in type 1 diabetes. Ophthalmology. 1998;105(10):1801–15.
4. Brown DM, Nguyen QD, Marcus DM, et al. Long-term outcomes of ranibizumab therapy for diabetic macular edema: the 36-month results from two phase III trials: RISE and RIDE. Ophthalmology. 2013;120(10):2013–22.
5. Diabetic Retinopathy Clinical Research Network, Elman MJ, Qin H, et al. Intravitreal ranibizumab for diabetic macular edema with prompt versus deferred laser treatment: three-year randomized trial results. Ophthalmology. 2012;119(11):2312–8.
6. Diabetic Retinopathy Clinical Research Network, Googe J, Brucker AJ, et al. Randomized trial evaluating short-term effects of intravitreal ranibizumab or triamcinolone acetonide on macular edema after focal/grid laser for diabetic macular edema in eyes also receiving panretinal photocoagulation. Retina Phila Pa. 2011;31(6):1009–27.
7. Do DV, Nguyen QD, Boyer D, et al. One-year outcomes of the da Vinci Study of VEGF Trap-Eye in eyes with diabetic macular edema. Ophthalmology. 2012;119(8):1658–65.
8. Mitchell P, Bandello F, Schmidt-Erfurth U, et al. The RESTORE study: ranibizumab monotherapy or combined with laser versus laser monotherapy for diabetic macular edema. Ophthalmology. 2011;118(4):615–25.
9. Massin P, Bandello F, Garweg JG, et al. Safety and efficacy of ranibizumab in diabetic macular edema (RESOLVE Study): a 12-month, randomized, controlled, double-masked, multicenter phase II study. Diabetes Care. 2010;33(11):2399–405.
10. Nguyen QD, Brown DM, Marcus DM, et al. Ranibizumab for diabetic macular edema: results from 2 phase III randomized trials: RISE and RIDE. Ophthalmology. 2012;119(4):789–801.
11. Nguyen QD, Shah SM, Heier JS, et al. Primary end point (six months) results of the ranibizumab for edema of the mAcula in diabetes (READ-2) study. Ophthalmology. 2009;116(11):2175–2181.e1.
12. Nguyen QD, Shah SM, Khwaja AA, et al. Two-year outcomes of the ranibizumab for edema of the mAcula in diabetes (READ-2) study. Ophthalmology. 2010;117(11):2146–51.
13. Regillo CD, Brown GC, Savino PJ, et al. Diabetic papillopathy. Patient characteristics and fundus findings. Arch Ophthalmol. 1995;113(7):889–95.
14. Hayreh SS, Zimmerman MB. Nonarteritic anterior ischemic optic neuropathy: clinical characteristics in diabetic patients versus nondiabetic patients. Ophthalmology. 2008;115(10):1818–25.
15. Al-Haddad CE, Jurdi FA, Bashshur ZF. Intravitreal triamcinolone acetonide for the management of diabetic papillopathy. Am J Ophthalmol. 2004;137(6):1151–3.
16. Al-Hinai AS, Al-Abri MS, Al-Hajri RH. Diabetic papillopathy with macular edema treated with intravitreal bevacizumab. Oman J Ophthalmol. 2011;4(3):135–8.
17. Kim M, Lee J-H, Lee S-J. Diabetic papillopathy with macular edema treated with intravitreal ranibizumab. Clin OphthalmolAuckl NZ. 2013;7:2257–60.

Optical Coherence Tomography of Vascular Disorders, Malformations, and Tumors

4

Margaret A. Greven and Craig M. Greven

Abstract

Optical coherence tomography (OCT), in conjunction with clinical examination, has become an important imaging modality to aid in both the diagnosis and treatment of ocular disorders. In this chapter, specific OCT
findings of a variety of vascular diseases of the retina, choroid, and optic
nerve are described through real clinical cases.

Keywords

Optical coherence tomography • Branch retinal vein occlusion • Central
retinal vein occlusion • Branch retinal artery occlusion • Central retinal
artery occlusion • Ophthalmic artery occlusion • Choroidal infarction •
Purtscher's retinopathy • Arteritic ischemic optic neuropathy • Nonarteritic ischemic optic neuropathy • Retinal arterial macroaneurysm •
Valsalva retinopathy • Radiation retinopathy • Macular telangiectasia •
Coats disease • Polypoidal • Central serous chorioretinopathy • Retinopathy
of prematurity • FEVR • Cavernous hemangioma • Retinal hemangioblastoma • Racemose hemangioma • Choroidal hemangioma

Introduction

Vascular diseases and malformations of the retina, choroid, and optic nerve represent a large
portion of pathology seen in everyday practice by
all ophthalmologists. Previously, modalities used
to evaluate these entities included ophthalmoscopy, intravenous fluorescein angiography, and
indocyanine green angiography (ICG). In the last
10 years, optical coherence tomography (OCT)
has become the primary tool used as an adjunct to

M.A. Greven, MD (✉) • C.M. Greven, MD
Department of Ophthalmology, Wills Eye Hospital,
Philadelphia, PA, USA
e-mail: margaret.greven@gmail.com;
cgreven@wakehealth.edu

© Springer International Publishing Switzerland 2016
A. Girach, R.C. Sergott (eds.), *Optical Coherence Tomography*,
DOI 10.1007/978-3-319-24817-2_4

clinical examination for the diagnosis and management of ocular vascular diseases and malformations. This chapter describes, through real clinical cases, OCT features of a variety of diseases of the retina, optic nerve, and choroid.

Retinal and Choroidal Vascular Occlusive Disorders

Branch Retinal Vein Occlusion

Case 1
A 55-year-old obese man with history of myocardial infarction and hypertension presented with acute blurring of vision and a superior visual field cut in the left eye. The vision in the affected left eye was 20/100 (Fig. 4.1).

Case 2
A 68-year-old female with non-insulin-dependent diabetes mellitus and hypertension presented with acute blurring of vision in the left eye. Visual acuity in the affected eye was 20/80 (Fig. 4.2).

Case 3
A 70-year-old female with hypertension and hyperlipidemia presented with diminished vision in the right eye. At presentation, her visual acuity in the affected eye was count fingers at 3 feet (Fig. 4.3).

Macular edema commonly occurs and is the major reason for decreased visual acuity associated with branch retinal vein occlusion [1]. OCT readily demonstrates this cystoid macular edema and enables monitoring of response to therapy such as intravitreal VEGF or steroid injections [2–5]. Serous retinal detachment, as well as disruption of the IS-OS junction and external limiting membrane, is also frequently demonstrated by OCT in BRVO [2–4]. Some of these OCT features, particularly IS-OS integrity

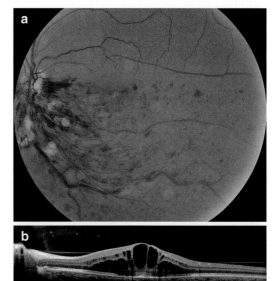

Fig. 4.1 (**a**) A fundus photo of the patient's left eye demonstrates a branch retinal vein occlusion (BRVO). Numerous intraretinal hemorrhages, cotton wool spots, and dilated, tortuous vessels along the inferior arcade are noted. (**b**) An OCT horizontally oriented through the patient's macula at presentation, demonstrating macular edema with cystic fluid in multiple levels of the retina

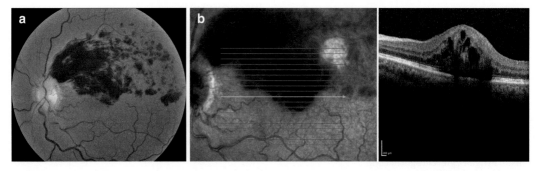

Fig. 4.2 (**a**) A fundus photo of the affected left eye demonstrating a BRVO along the superior arcade. There are flame hemorrhages and dot-blot hemorrhages in the superior macula. (**b**) A horizontally oriented OCT through the patient's macula demonstrates cystic fluid mostly within the outer retinal layers

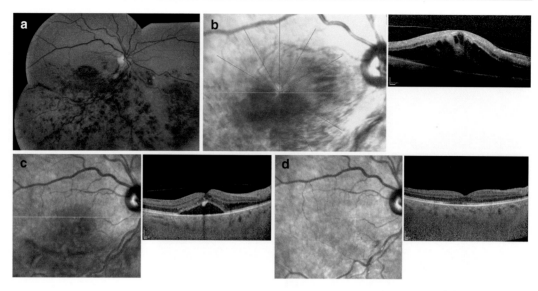

Fig. 4.3 (**a**) Fundus photo shows a hemiretinal vein occlusion (HRVO) with numerous intraretinal hemorrhages in the inferior half of the retina. (**b**) A horizontally oriented macular OCT at presentation, with cystic fluid in the outer retinal layers and subretinal fluid. (**c**) OCT at 1 month after initial presentation, demonstrating resolution of cystic intraretinal fluid with development of exudates within deeper retinal layers and persistent subretinal fluid. (**d**) An OCT 1 year after presentation after the patient was treated with intravitreal Avastin, demonstrating resolution of subretinal fluid as well as temporal macular retinal nerve fiber layer thinning and disruption of the inner segment-outer segment junction (IS-OS junction) temporal to the fovea; visual acuity improved to 20/30 after treatment

and external limiting membrane status, may predict final visual acuity in patients with BRVO [5]. Chronically, sectoral retinal nerve fiber layer thinning can be seen on OCT in the previously involved retina [6].

BRVO: Summary of OCT characteristics

- Cystoid macular edema
- Serous retinal detachment
- IS-OS disruption
- External limiting membrane disruption
- Chronically, sectoral nerve fiber layer thinning

Central Retinal Vein Occlusion

Case 4
A 68-year-old female presented with acute vision loss in the left eye, with visual acuity of 20/200 (Fig. 4.4).

Case 5
A 55-year-old man with type two diabetes mellitus and hyperlipidemia presented with acute loss of vision in his right eye, with visual acuity of 20/400 (Fig. 4.5).

Case 6
A 63-year-old female with hypertension and rheumatoid arthritis presented with acute change in vision in the left eye which occurred acutely 3 days prior. On examination, she was 20/25 in the unaffected right eye and 20/30 in the affected left eye (Fig. 4.6).

As with branch retinal vein occlusions, central retinal vein occlusions can often result in cystoid macular edema [7–9]. These spaces can be seen in all retinal layers and can also be combined with serous retinal detachment [8]. Central retinal thickness on OCT tends to be thicker in ischemic CRVO than nonischemic CRVO and may help predict ultimate visual prognosis in patients presenting with this condition [8]. CRVO can result in disruption of the IS-OS junction and/or loss of inner retinal layers on OCT, both of which portend a worse visual prognosis [8, 9].

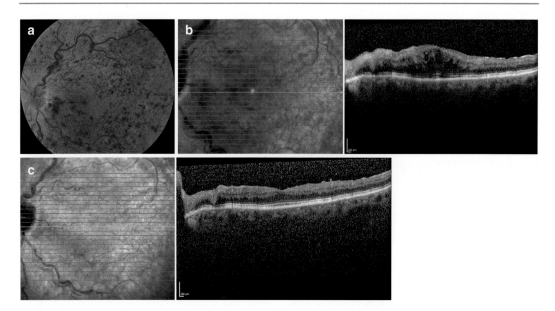

Fig. 4.4 (**a**) A fundus photograph of the affected eye shows dilated and tortuous retinal arteries and veins, optic disk edema, and numerous intraretinal hemorrhages, consistent with a central retinal vein occlusion (CRVO). (**b**) A horizontal OCT through the macula confirms the presence of macular edema involving mostly the inner retinal layers. (**c**) An OCT 3 months after intravitreal Avastin injection shows resolution of edema and generalized retinal thinning

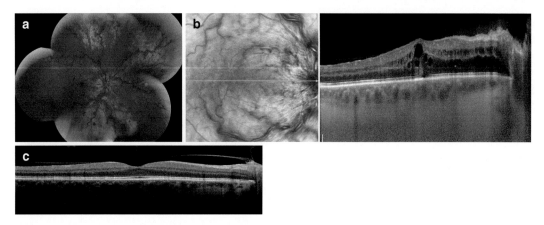

Fig. 4.5 (**a**) Fundus photo demonstrates findings consistent with a CRVO: dilated tortuous veins, nerve fiber layer hemorrhages, and optic nerve swelling. (**b**) A horizontally oriented macular OCT shows cystoid macular edema. (**c**) Resolution of macular edema after intravitreal VEGF treatment

CRVO: Summary of OCT characteristics

- Cystoid macular edema
- Serous retinal detachment
- Acutely, retinal thickening
- Hemorrhage in multiple retinal layers
- Defect of IS-OS line
- Loss of inner retinal layers

Branch Retinal Artery Occlusion

Case 7

A 78-year-old obese man with hypertension, hyperlipidemia, and diabetes mellitus presented with acute loss of vision in the right eye, with visual acuity of 20/400 (Fig. 4.7).

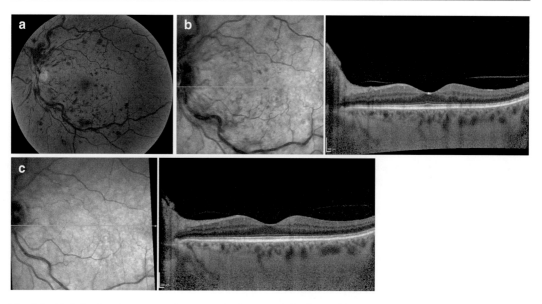

Fig. 4.6 (**a**) A fundus photograph of the left eye shows findings consistent with CRVO. (**b**) A horizontally oriented macular OCT at presentation, showing mild retinal thickening of the inner retinal layers. (**c**) An OCT 6 months later without treatment shows improvement in previously seen thickening

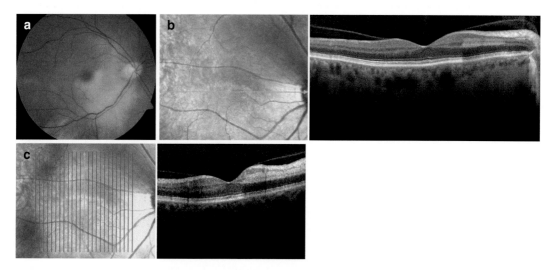

Fig. 4.7 (**a**) A fundus photograph of the affected eye demonstrates inferior retinal whitening consistent with branch retinal artery occlusion (BRAO). (**b**) A horizontally oriented OCT through the macula demonstrates increased inner retina reflectivity near the nerve, with more normal contour through the temporal aspect of the macula. (**c**) Vertically oriented OCT through the macula allows comparison of the normal superior retina with the involved inferior retina, which displays relatively increased reflectivity and thickness in the inner retinal layers with corresponding decreased reflectivity in the outer retinal layers

Case 8

A 72-year-old man with atrial fibrillation and hypertension presented with acute painless vision loss and changes in his superior visual field. The vision in the affected left eye is 20/400 (Fig. 4.8).

BRAO occurs as a result of embolization, thrombosis, or vasospasm and results in acute, painless loss of vision in the visual field corresponding to the obstructed artery [10]. OCT of acute BRAO demonstrates thickening of the

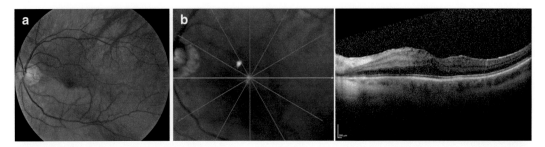

Fig. 4.8 (**a**) Fundus photo shows inferior retinal whitening and yellow plaque in the vessel at the disk consistent with BRAO. There is also incidentally a choroidal nevus. (**b**) OCT through the fovea shows increased reflectivity and thickness in the inner retinal layers, particularly of the involved nasal aspect of the macula, with more preserved retinal architecture of the temporal aspect of the macula

neurosensory retina resulting from intracellular edema in the inner retinal layers [10–13]. Acutely, the inner retinal layers also have increased reflectivity on OCT, and the photoreceptor and retinal pigment epithelium show corresponding hyporeflectivity as a result of shadowing effect [10–13]. A prominent middle limiting membrane sign, defined as a hyperreflective line at the inner part of the outer plexiform layer, may be noted on OCT in BRAO or CRAO acutely and can persist longer than the aforementioned signs, up to 1 month after onset of symptoms [13]. Late findings on OCT include retinal atrophy and indiscriminate inner retinal layers [13].

BRAO: Summary of OCT findings

- Acute
  - Inner retinal edema and hyperreflectivity
  - Outer retina hyporeflectivity
  - Prominent middle limiting membrane
- Chronic
  - Retinal atrophy with loss of inner retinal layers

Central Retinal Artery Occlusion

Case 9

A 70-year-old man developed acute decrease in vision in his left eye, with visual acuity on presentation of count fingers at one foot (Fig. 4.9).

Case 10

A 60-year-old woman with hypertension and hyperlipidemia with acute loss of vision in the left eye upon awakening, with visual acuity of count fingers at one foot (Fig. 4.10).

Central retinal artery occlusions share many OCT features in common with BRAOs. Acutely, they demonstrate thickening and hyperreflectivity of the inner retina with shadowing effect and thus hyporeflectivity of the photoreceptors and retinal pigment epithelium [13–15]. The prominent middle limiting membrane may also be seen in OCT of central retinal artery occlusions and may last longer than the aforementioned signs [13]. Chronically, the inner retinal layers are thinned and atrophied resulting in loss of discrimination on OCT of the inner retinal layers [13–15]. Increased foveal thickness at presentation on OCT or at final follow-up on OCT are correlated with poorer visual prognosis [15].

CRAO: Summary of OCT findings

- Thickening of inner retina
- Hyperreflectivity of inner retina
- Corresponding decreased reflectivity of outer retina/RPE

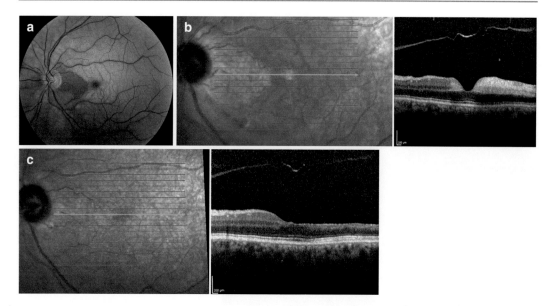

Fig. 4.9 (**a**) Fundus photo shows retinal whitening with classic cherry red spot and sparing of the retina in the distribution of the cilioretinal artery. (**b**) Horizontally oriented OCT through the macula at presentation shows hyperreflectivity and edema of the outer retina and retinal thickening at the fovea and temporal aspect of the macula sparing the nasal retina supplied by the cilioretinal artery. (**c**) OCT through macula 4 months later shows atrophy of inner retinal layers in the involved retina

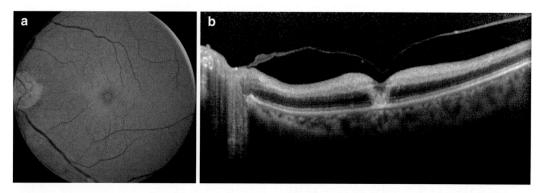

Fig. 4.10 (**a**) Fundus photo of the affected eye shows retinal whitening and cherry red spot consistent with CRAO. (**b**) Horizontally oriented OCT through the macula at presentation shows edema and hyperreflectivity of inner retinal layers with relative shadowing of the outer retinal layers

Ophthalmic Artery Occlusion

Case 11

A 54-year-old female underwent craniotomy for resection of a frontal lobe meningioma. Upon awakening from surgery, her vision was no light perception in her left eye. There was a 4+ afferent pupillary defect (Fig. 4.11).

Ophthalmic artery occlusion imaged by OCT demonstrates diffuse edema of the retina. There is hyperreflectivity of all layers of the retina on OCT but loss of the inner segment-outer segment junction line and thinning of the retinal nerve fiber layer [16]. Chronically, atrophy of all layers of the neurosensory retina occurs.

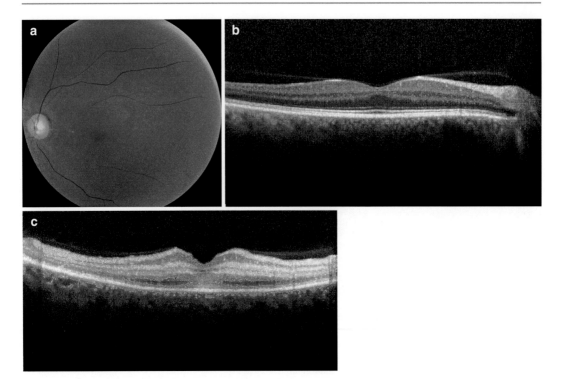

Fig. 4.11 (**a**) Fundus photo demonstrates a pale optic nerve, arterial and venous attenuation, and dusky retinal appearance. (**b**) A horizontally oriented OCT through the unaffected right eye. (**c**) By comparison, the OCT from the affected left eye demonstrates diffuse retinal edema, hyperreflectivity of the all retinal layers, and decreased retinal nerve fiber layer thickness. OCT also demonstrates lack of photoreceptors in the inner and outer segment line

Ophthalmic artery occlusion: Summary of OCT characteristics

- Acutely show retinal edema
- Thinning of retinal nerve fiber layer
- Loss of IS-OS junction
- Later develop atrophy and thinning of all retinal layers

Choroidal Infarction

Case 12

A 39-year-old woman with decreased vision in the right eye greater than left eye for 4 months. She was recently hospitalized in the intensive care unit after overdosing on prescription drugs, and her course was complicated by diffuse intravascular coagulation. She has had poor vision since her hospital stay. On presentation, her acuity was count fingers at 3 ft in the right eye and 20/50 in the left eye (Fig. 4.12).

Choroidal infarction has multiple causes including vascular conditions such as elevated blood pressure, eclampsia, or hypercoagulability; inflammatory conditions such as giant cell arteritis; autoimmune conditions such as Wegener's; or trauma [17–20]. Optical coherence findings in choroidal infarction include thinning of the retina and choroid along with a lumpy hyperreflectivity in the choroid and RPE.

Choroidal infarction: Summary of OCT characteristics

- Atrophy of inner retinal layers
- Thinning and atrophy of choroid
- Hyperreflectivity and nodular appearance to RPE/inner choroid

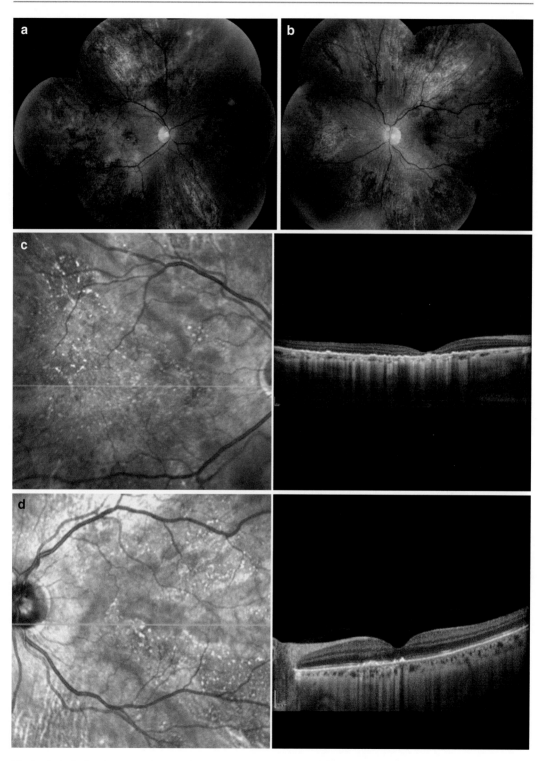

Fig. 4.12 (**a, b**) Fundus photos of the right eye and left eye show wedge-shaped infarcts of the retinal pigment epithelium and outer retina. (**c, d**) Horizontally oriented OCTs through the macula of the right eye and left eyes. The patient's right eye, with worse vision, demonstrates severe thinning of the retina and choroid along with a lumpy hyperreflectivity in the choroid underlying the macula, thus accounting for this eye's poorer vision. In the left eye, the foveal architecture is relatively preserved with some distortion in the RPE, resulting in better visual acuity in that eye

Ischemic Optic Neuropathies

Non-arteritic Ischemic Optic Neuropathy

Case 13

A 57-year-old man with history of non-arteritic ischemic optic neuropathy (NAION) in his left eye 10 years prior, hypertension, and obstructive sleep apnea, who noted sudden-onset vision loss in the right eye upon awakening. His visual acuity in the affected eye was 20/40, and it was 20/30 in the previously affected left eye. He had an inferior visual field cut in the newly affected eye. His exam was notable for a swollen hyperemic disk in the right eye (Fig. 4.13).

NAION is thought to result from transient hypoperfusion to the optic nerve resulting from a crowded optic nerve head, or the "disk at risk." It is characterized by sudden and painless vision loss with optic nerve edema. Optic nerve OCT in NAION will acutely demonstrate segmental optic nerve edema. In the fellow eye, a small cup-to-disk ratio may be noted on OCT and may serve to help confirm the diagnosis of NAION. Chronically, months after initial event when edema is resolved, OCT can be used to demonstrate retinal nerve fiber layer thinning at the involved aspect of the optic nerve [20, 21].

NAION: Summary of OCT characteristics

- Acutely optic nerve edema
- Small cup-to-disk ratio in the fellow eye
- Chronically, retinal nerve fiber layer thinning

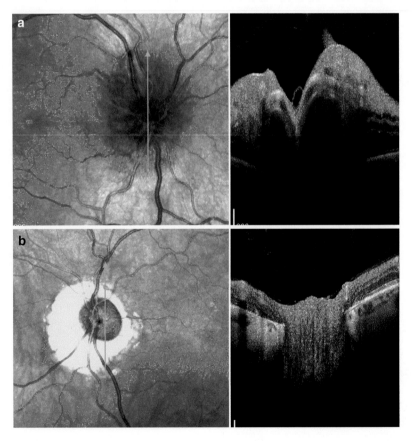

Fig. 4.13 (**a**) OCT of the right optic nerve demonstrates optic nerve edema and increased peripapillary retinal nerve fiber layer thickness. (**b**) Optic nerve OCT of the left eye: there is decreased thickness of the peripapillary retinal nerve fiber layer in all quadrants except temporally

Arteritic Ischemic Optic Neuropathy

Case 14

A 64-year-old female presented with graying vision in the right eye, temporal headaches, jaw claudication, myalgias, and fevers. Her visual acuity in the affected right eye was 20/60 and was 20/20 in the unaffected eye. There was an afferent pupillary defect in the right eye. Her erythrocyte sedimentation rate, C-reactive protein, and platelets were elevated. The patient was initiated on intravenous steroids and underwent a temporal artery biopsy, yielding a positive result and thus was diagnosed with arteritic ischemic optic neuropathy. Her symptoms resolved secondary to prompt steroid treatment (Fig. 4.14).

Giant cell arteritis is a vasculitis that most often results in vision loss due to arteritic ischemic optic neuropathy. Patients with giant cell arteritis may present with visual symptoms such as blurry vision due to AION or CRAO, or diplopia. Affected individuals may also have systemic symptoms such as malaise, temporal tenderness, jaw claudication, fevers, or myalgias. Acutely, AION is characterized by chalky white pallor of the optic nerve, which is readily demonstrated by OCT. Chronically, there is atrophy and thinning of the peripapillary retinal nerve fiber layer, also demonstrable by OCT.

AION: Summary of OCT characteristics

- Acutely, optic nerve edema
- Chronically, retinal nerve fiber layer atrophy

Miscellaneous Acquired Retinal Vascular Diseases

Retinal Arterial Macroaneurysm

Case 15

A 73-year-old female with hypertension and hyperlipidemia presents with acute worsening of vision in her right eye. On presentation in the office, her blood pressure is 210/110. Her visual acuity is 20/50 in the affected right eye and 20/25 in the unaffected left eye (Fig. 4.15).

Retinal arterial macroaneurysm (RAM) is an acquired focal area of dilation of the retinal arterial wall. This focal vascular abnormality has abnormal permeability and can result in macular edema, serous retinal detachment, and hard exudation (intraretinal lipid accumulation). Rupture of the aneurysm can result in retinal hemorrhage in multiple retinal layers, subretinal hemorrhage, or vitreous hemorrhage [22–24]. OCT may demonstrate this macular edema with retinal fluid typically involving the outer retinal layers; it may

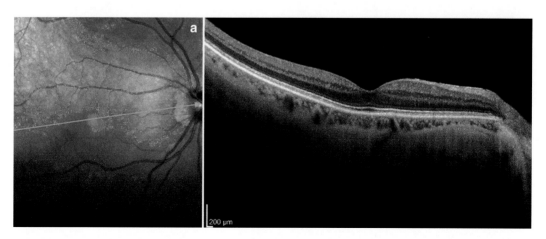

Fig. 4.14 (**a**) A horizontally oriented OCT of the patient's right macula 2 weeks after initial presentation demonstrating normal retinal architecture and lack of optic nerve edema. (**b**) The peripapillary retinal nerve fiber layer map for the right and the left eyes. There is borderline thinning of the RNFL superiorly and nasally in the affected right eye. Incidentally, there is thinning of the nasal RNFL in the unaffected left eye

b

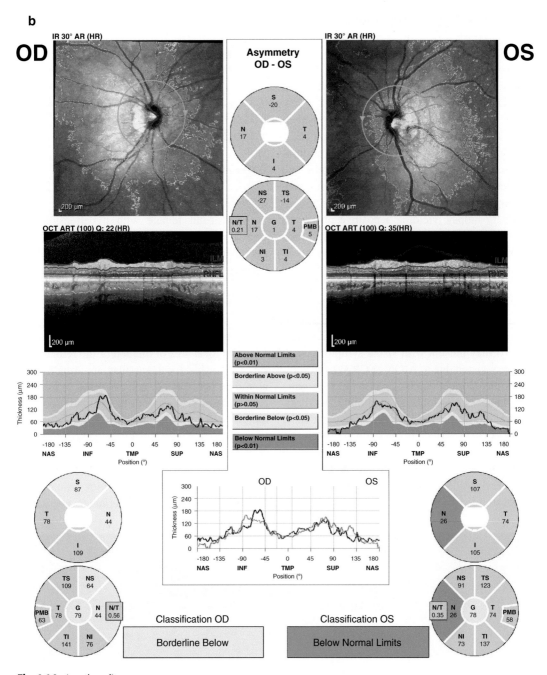

Fig. 4.14 (continued)

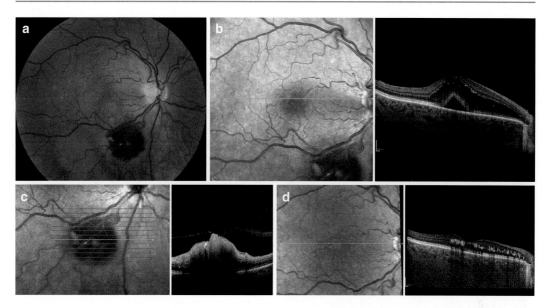

Fig. 4.15 (**a**) The patient's fundus photo, demonstrating subretinal hemorrhage along the inferior arcade and a retinal arterial macroaneurysm (RAM). (**b**) A horizontally oriented OCT through the patient's macula, demonstrating intraretinal hard exudates, retinal edema, and subretinal fluid, accounting for the patient's decreased vision. (**c**) An OCT through the macroaneurysm itself, demonstrating elevation and hyperreflectivity of the overlying retina and shadowing of the deeper retinal layers. (**d**) A horizontally oriented macular OCT 3 months later, showing resolution of subretinal fluid and more numerous hard exudates

also demonstrate preretinal, intraretinal, or subretinal hemorrhage [22, 24]. Serous retinal detachment with subretinal fluid can also be demonstrated on OCT [22, 25]. With resolution of the intraretinal fluid, OCT can demonstrate increases in exudates within the outer plexiform layer [23]. OCT of the macroaneurysm itself shows round inner retinal elevation of the internal limiting membrane and ganglion cell layers with underlying shadowing [23, 24]. Occasionally, OCT may show subretinal fluid beneath the macroaneurysm [24]. An unruptured aneurysm may be seen on OCT as a small area of hyperintensity with underlying lower intensity lumen producing shadowing of the deeper retinal layers [26].

Retinal arterial macroaneurysm: Summary of OCT features

- RAM appears as dome-shaped elevation of the retina with shadowing
- May be accompanied with subretinal fluid
- After resolution of subretinal fluid, hard exudates develop

Radiation Retinopathy

Case 16

A 60-year-old man with history of left frontal lobe tumor status posttreatment with chemotherapy and external beam radiation 18 months prior to presentation. On presentation he described a decline in his vision in the left eye over the last 2 months. His visual acuity was 20/100 in the affected left eye and there was a left relative afferent pupillary defect (Fig. 4.16).

Radiation retinopathy can be a result of radiation treatment to the head and neck or plaque radiotherapy to the eye. It is characterized by an ischemic maculopathy. Optical coherence tomography can demonstrate changes of radiation retinopathy prior to clinical symptoms and thus facilitate its prompt treatment [27]. Classic OCT findings include intraretinal cystic fluid, thinning of the ganglion cell layer, retinal atrophy, and hard exudates [27–30].

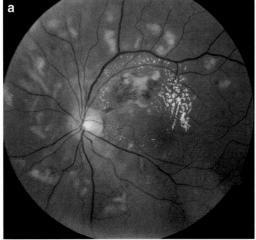

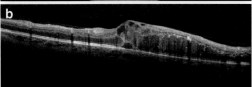

Fig. 4.16 (**a**) Fundus photograph, with multiple cotton wool spots, hard exudates within the macula, and flame-shaped hemorrhages consistent with a BRAO along the superior aspect of the macula. (**b**) Horizontally oriented OCT through the macula shows retinal edema with cystic fluid in multiple retinal layers, retinal atrophy, and hard exudates in the outer plexiform layer

Radiation retinopathy: Summary of OCT characteristics

- Cystic intraretinal fluid
- Macular edema
- Hard exudates
- Atrophy

Purtscher's Retinopathy

Case 17

A 28-year-old male who was in a motor vehicle accident resulting in bilateral rib fractures and pulmonary contusions complained of decreased vision in both eyes following the accident. On presentation, he had count fingers vision at three feet in both eyes (Fig. 4.17).

Purtscher's retinopathy was initially described in 1910 by Otmar Purtscher in a patient with severe head trauma [31]. Purtscher's has also been described in other conditions including pancreatitis, compressive injury to the thorax, long bone fractures, childbirth, collagen vascular disease, and hemolytic uremic syndrome [32–34]. Early optical coherence tomography features of Purtscher's retinopathy include irregular edema and hyperreflectivity of the ganglion cell layer, shadowing and hyporeflectivity of the deeper retinal layers, and cystic macular edema. Chronically, OCT of the retina shows atrophy and loss of distinct retinal layers and loss of normal foveal contour.

Purtscher's retinopathy: Summary of OCT characteristics

- Acute: thickening and hyperreflectivity of the ganglion cell layer
- Chronic: retinal atrophy

Idiopathic Macular Telangiectasia

Case 18

A 44-year-old female presented with type 2 diabetes mellitus who noted blank areas in her vision in both eyes when reading which has been progressive over the last 4–5 weeks. Her visual acuity is 20/20 in the right eye and 20/50 in the left eye (Fig. 4.18).

Macular telangiectasia type 2A is a bilateral disorder of Muller's cells resulting in telangiectatic and leaky capillaries within the fovea. This condition can result in cystic intraretinal fluid, thinning and disruption of the IS-OS junction, and foveal atrophy; all features can readily be identified on OCT images [35–37].

Macular telangiectasia: Summary of OCT characteristics

- Cystic intraretinal fluid
- Thinning and disruption of the IS-OS junction
- Foveal atrophy

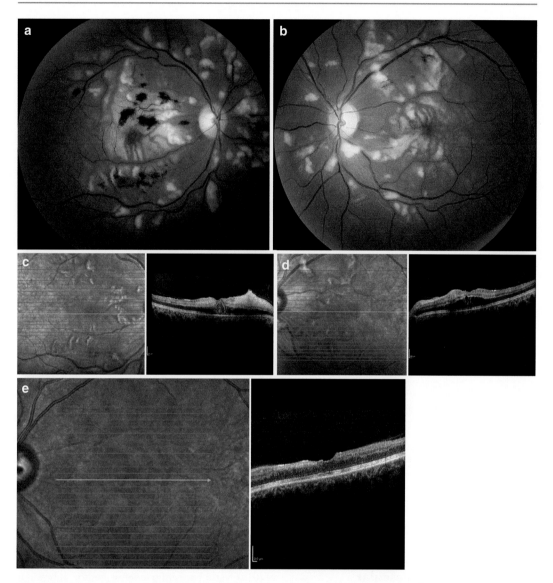

Fig. 4.17 Fundus photos of the right (**a**) and left (**b**) eyes demonstrate multiple bilateral cotton wool spots and intraretinal hemorrhages in the right eye more than the left eye consistent with Purtscher's retinopathy. OCT of the right (**c**) and left (**d**) eye on presentation shows irregular edema and hyperreflectivity of the ganglion cell layer, shadowing and hyporeflectivity of the deeper retinal layers, and cystoid macular edema. (**e**) The patient's OCT of the left eye 3 months later demonstrates retinal atrophy

Valsalva Retinopathy

Case 19

A 30-year-old otherwise healthy female presented with acute onset of vision loss in the left eye after an episode of coughing. Her vision loss was stable since onset. In the right eye, her vision was 20/20, and in the affected left eye, it was 20/400 (Fig. 4.19).

Valsalva retinopathy presents as sudden vision loss caused by premacular hemorrhage related to Valsalva maneuver. OCT of Valsalva retinopathy demonstrates dome-shaped sub-ILM hemorrhage, subhyaloid hemorrhage, or both [38–40].

Valsalva retinopathy: Summary of OCT characteristics

- Occurs after Valsalva maneuver: coughing or sneezing, bearing down, heavy lifting, playing musical instrument
- OCT demonstrates subhyaloid or subinternal limiting membrane hemorrhage

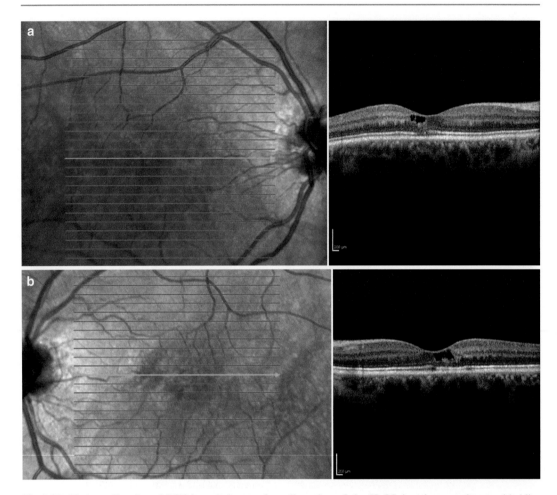

Fig. 4.18 Horizontally oriented OCT through the macula of the right (**a**) and left (**b**) eyes shows cystic intraretinal fluid involving the fovea of both eyes, with thinning and disruption of the IS-OS junction, consistent with idiopathic macular telangiectasia type 2A

Congenital Retinal Vascular Diseases

Retinopathy of Prematurity

Case 20

An 11-year-old girl with history of prematurity, born at 26 weeks with birth weight of 2.2 pounds. She had been noted to have retinopathy of prematurity (ROP) in infancy that had resolved without treatment. Her visual acuity was 20/25 in both eyes (Fig. 4.20).

OCT of patients born prematurely, even into adulthood, demonstrates either absence or shallowing of the foveal pit with persistence of inner retinal layers within the fovea [40–44]. This finding does not correlate with visual acuity potential

[40]. Cystoid macular edema and/or subretinal fluid may also be demonstrated on optical coherence tomography in patients with retinopathy of prematurity [41, 44].

ROP: Summary of OCT characteristics

- Loss of foveal contour
- Persistence of inner retinal layers
- Subretinal fluid
- Cystoid macular edema

Familial Exudative Vitreoretinopathy

Case 21

A 14-year-old male with reduced vision in his left eye for approximately one year. His visual

Fig. 4.19 (a) Fundus photograph of the affected eye demonstrates layering subhyaloid hemorrhage with sub-ILM hemorrhage overlying the fovea. (b) OCT of the involved eye shows bullous sub-ILM hemorrhage

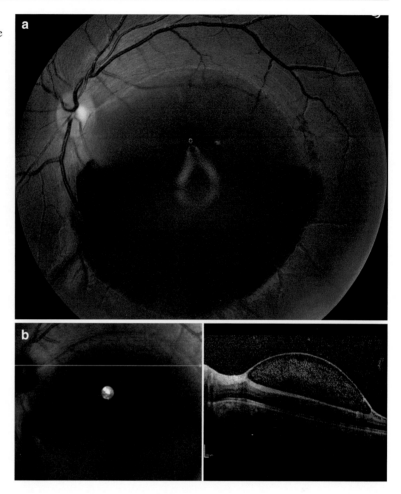

acuity in the right eye was 20/20 and in the left eye was 20/70. Fundoscopic examination of the right eye (not shown) demonstrated peripheral areas of nonperfusion (Fig. 4.21).

FEVR is a hereditary vitreoretinal disorder characterized by areas of peripheral retinal nonperfusion, neovascularization, exudation, and tractional retinal detachment. OCT features of FEVR include tractional retinal detachment, cystic intraretinal fluid, and preretinal or intraretinal exudates [45]. OCT may also demonstrate areas of vitreoretinal adhesion contributing to decreased vision in this condition [46].

FEVR: Summary of OCT characteristics

- Tractional retinal detachment
- Intraretinal fluid
- Preretinal or intraretinal exudates
- Vitreoretinal adhesion

Coats Disease

Case 22

An 8-year-old male presented with chronically poor vision in the right eye and normal vision in the unaffected left eye. His visual acuity in the affected right eye is count fingers at three feet (Fig. 4.22).

Coats disease is a unilateral congenital condition characterized by abnormal telangiectatic and aneurysmal changes resulting in the accumulation of intraretinal and subretinal hard exudates. It occurs most often unilaterally in young males under 5 years of age. Frequently,

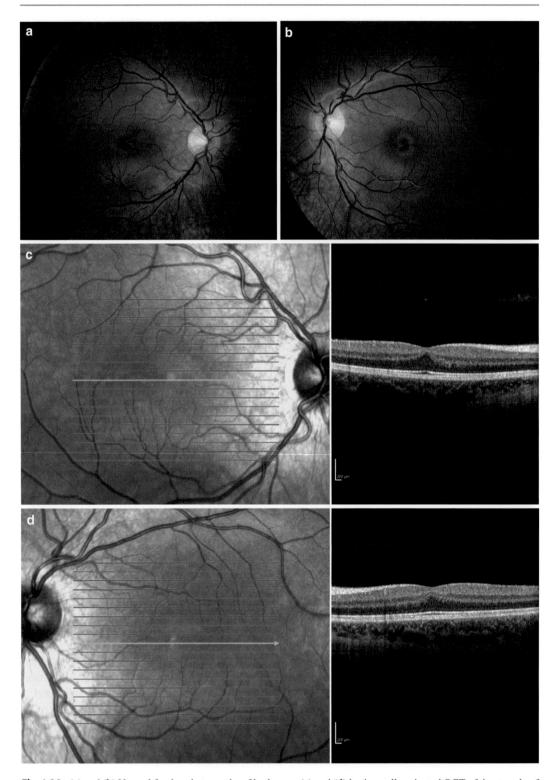

Fig. 4.20 (**a**) and (**b**) Normal fundus photographs of both eyes. (**c**) and (**d**) horizontally oriented OCT of the macula of both eyes shows flattening of the foveal contour and loss of foveal depression

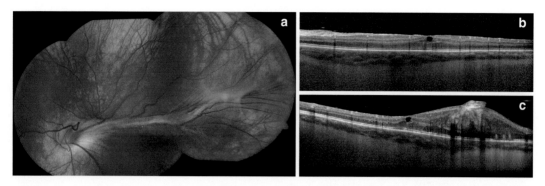

Fig. 4.21 (**a**) Fundus photo of the left eye demonstrates temporal dragging of the retina. Clinically, the patient was noted to have peripheral nonperfusion and neovascularization in the left eye. (**b**) Horizontally oriented OCT through the fovea shows relatively atrophic retina with cystic intraretinal fluid at the fovea. (**c**) Vertically oriented OCT through the fovea again demonstrates this cystic intraretinal fluid and shows the temporally dragged retina as an elevated and disorganized mound with loss of normal retinal architecture. The patient was diagnosed with familial exudative vitreoretinopathy (FEVR)

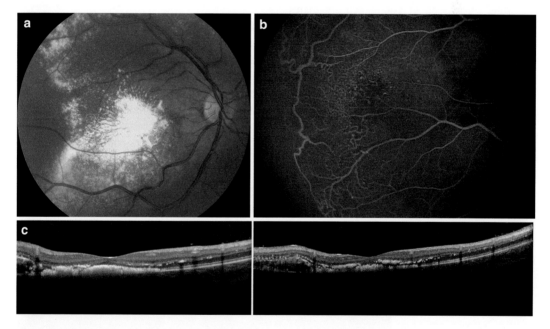

Fig. 4.22 (**a**) Demonstrates dense hard exudates within the macula and fluorescein angiography; (**b**) shows vascular findings consistent with a diagnosis of Coats disease. (**c**) A horizontal OCT through the macula and (**d**) is a vertical OCT through the macula. Both OCT cuts demonstrate dense subfoveal and juxtafoveal hard exudates, a hallmark of Coats disease

the condition may lead to exudative retinal detachment. OCT demonstrates these exudates readily and can also demonstrate areas of retinal detachment [47, 48].

Coats Disease: Summary of OCT characteristics

- Intraretinal and subretinal hard exudates
- Exudative retinal detachment

Choroidal Vascular Diseases

Central Serous Chorioretinopathy

Case 23

A 55-year-old man with hypertension presented with metamorphopsia and decreased vision in his left eye. He has had multiple episodes of similar symptoms in the past in the affected eye and has been diagnosed with chronic central serous chorioretinopathy (CSCR). His visual acuity in the right eye is 20/25 and is 20/50 in the affected left eye. Examination showed subretinal fluid in the left eye (Fig. 4.23).

CSCR is characterized by neurosensory retinal detachment with variable height of subretinal fluid, often seen in young healthy males. Patients may also frequently develop small detachments of the RPE corresponding with areas of leakage on fluorescein angiography [49–52]. OCT demonstrates that the photoreceptor outer segments elongate in the area of the neurosensory retinal detachment. In patients with chronic disease, intraretinal fluid and cystoid edema may occur [51]. The thickness of the outer nuclear layer (OPL) on OCT correlates with visual acuity in patients with CSCR, with patients having thinner ONL having poorer visual prognosis [51]. The integrity of the IS-OS junction also correlates with visual acuity. Patients with long-standing disease can develop retinal atrophy.

CSCR: Summary of OCT characteristics

- Subretinal fluid, pigment epithelial detachment
- Elongation of outer segments of photoreceptors
- Thickened choroid on enhanced depth imaging
- Chronically, retinal atrophy, thinning of OPL, and disruption of IS-OS junction

Polypoidal Choroidal Vasculopathy

Case 24

A 46-year-old male who noted a "veil over" his right eye upon awakening 3 months prior. On presentation, his visual acuity was 20/400 in the affected right eye and 20/25 in the left eye. He had a relative afferent pupillary defect in the right eye (Fig. 4.24).

PCV is a condition with abnormal choroidal vasculature resulting in hemorrhagic or serous detachment of the retinal pigment epithelium. OCT readily demonstrates these pigment epithelial detachments, often seen as dome-like elevations of the RPE. The polypoidal lesions are seen as characteristic hyperreflectivity beneath the RPE [53–55].

Polypoidal choroidal vasculopathy: Summary of OCT characteristics

- Choroidal vascular abnormality
- Dome-like elevation RPE and the neurosensory retina
  - Nodular appearance of choroid with characteristic hyperreflectivity

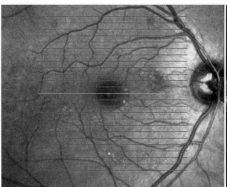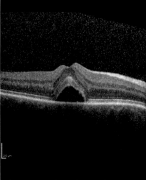

Fig. 4.23 A horizontally oriented macular OCT of the left eye demonstrates subfoveal fluid, ragged-appearing photoreceptor layer in the detached aspect of the retina, and a small focus of sub-RPE fluid

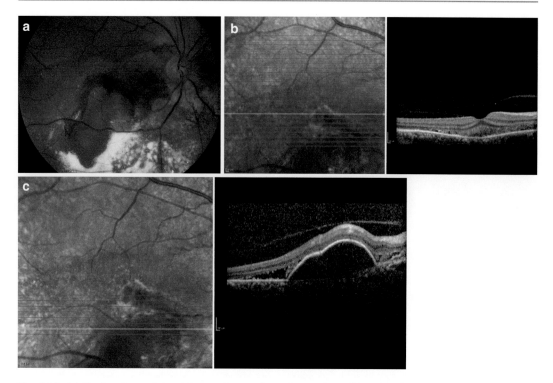

Fig. 4.24 (**a**) Fundus photo of the right eye shows sub-RPE and subretinal macular hemorrhage with exudation and pigment epithelial detachment. (**b**) and (**c**) OCT shows dome-like elevation of the retinal pigment epithelium with a nodular sub-RPE appearance and hyperreflectivity

Vascular Tumors

Cavernous Hemangioma of the Retina

Case 25

A 29-year-old female incidentally noted to have vascular mass in her right eye. She was asymptomatic on presentation and had 20/20 vision in both eyes (Fig. 4.25).

Cavernous hemangioma is a benign vascular hamartoma characterized by clusters of intraretinal aneurysms described as "grapelike" lesions [56–58]. Optical coherence tomography of cavernous hemangioma demonstrates optically dense mass with lobulated surface with cystic appearance replacing the normal neurosensory retina [56–58]. Shadowing may be seen beneath the tumor, preventing visibility of deeper levels of the retina. Preretinal fibrosis related to prior vitreous hemorrhage from the lesion may also been seen [57].

Cavernous hemangioma: Summary of OCT characteristics

- Vascular tumor composed of thin-walled veins
- OCT shows optically dense mass with lobulated surface
- Cystic appearance or anterior reflectivity resulting in shadowing blunting visibility of deeper levels

Retinal Capillary Hemangioma

Case 26

A 32-year-old female noted to have vascular tumor on routine examination. She is asymptomatic with 20/20 vision in each eye. She has undergone brain MRI which was negative to rule out brain vascular malformation and thus does not carry a diagnosis of von Hippel-Lindau syndrome (Fig. 4.26).

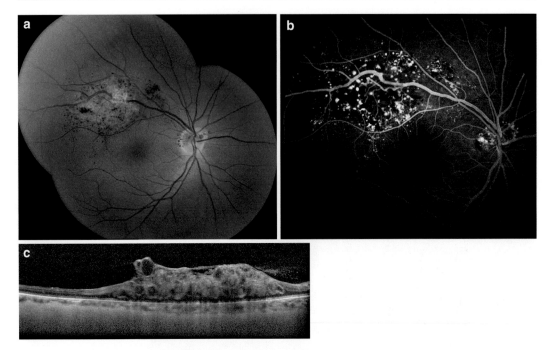

Fig. 4.25 (**a**) A fundus photo of the right eye shows a vascular tumor along the superior arcade with dark grape-like lesions within the retina, consistent with a cavernous hemangioma of the retina. (**b**) Fluorescein angiography of the affected eye shows numerous hyperfluorescent dot-like lesions in the corresponding area of the retina. (**c**) An OCT through the lesion shows lobulated cystic mass replacing the neurosensory retina

Retinal capillary hemangioma (retinal hemangioblastoma) is a vascular hamartoma of the retina characterized by an enlarged mass of hyperplastic capillaries fed by large feeder arteries and draining veins [57–59]. Optical coherence tomography of the tumor itself shows elevated inner retinal mass with posterior shadowing with disorganization of retinal layers within the lesion [57–59]. OCT may also demonstrate subretinal fluid, intraretinal edema, preretinal fibrosis, cystoid macular edema, and retinoschisis which may accompany this lesion [57, 59].

Retinal hemangioblastoma: Summary of OCT characteristics

- Retinal vascular tumor
- Optically dense inner retinal mass with posterior shadowing
- May demonstrate intra- or subretinal fluid
- May demonstrate macular edema

Racemose Hemangioma

Case 27

A 13-year-old male with decreased vision in the left eye and normal vision in the right eye. The vision in the affected eye is 20/200 (Fig. 4.27).

Racemose hemangioma is a congenital arteriovenous malformation (AVM) within the retina. It may occur in isolation or is associated with Wyburn-Mason syndrome in patients who also have AVM of the mandible, maxilla, midbrain, or pterygoid fossa. On OCT, this entity is shown as a cystic mass with underlying shadowing because of the dilated vessels [57].

Racemose hemangioma: Summary of OCT findings

- Intraretinal cystic mass
- Anterior reflectivity
- Rarely retinal atrophy, edema, and hemorrhage

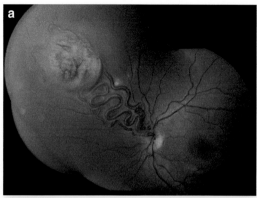

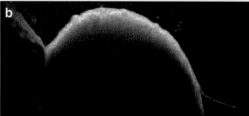

Fig. 4.26 (**a**) Composite fundus photograph demonstrates a red-orange mass in the superonasal aspect of the retina supplied by large dilated arteries and veins consistent with capillary hemangioma. (**b**) An OCT of the lesion, shows a dome-shaped mass elevating the retina and posterior shadowing

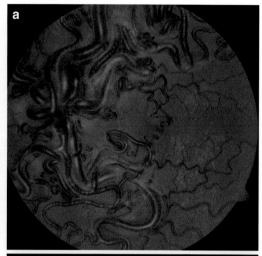

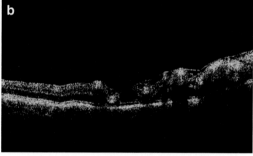

Fig. 4.27 (**a**) A fundus photo demonstrates dilated tortuous vessels consistent with racemose hemangioma, a type of congenital arteriovenous malformation. (**b**) Horizontally oriented OCT demonstrates intraretinal cystic mass

Choroidal Hemangioma

Case 28

A 12-year-old female with diagnosis of Sturge-Weber disease has port wine stain on left side of face, known glaucoma in the left eye s/p prior to glaucoma surgery. She has noted a decrease in her visual acuity in the left eye over the last few weeks. Her visual acuity in the right eye is 20/20 and in the affected left eye is 20/40 (Fig. 4.28).

Choroidal hemangioma is a choroidal vascular hamartoma that may be associated with Sturge-Weber syndrome. OCT findings of choroidal hemangioma include exudative retinal detachment, macular edema, subretinal fibrosis, and retinal atrophy [57, 58, 60]. The tumor itself

appears hyperreflective on its anterior surface but beneath this shows shadowing or decreased reflectivity compared to normal choroid appearance on OCT [57, 60].

Choroidal hemangioma: Summary of OCT characteristics

- Choroidal vascular tumor
- Anterior surface of tumor is hyperreflective on OCT with hyporeflectivity deeper in the tumor
- Retinal changes include retinal atrophy overlying the tumor, foveal cystoid edema, and/or subfoveal fluid

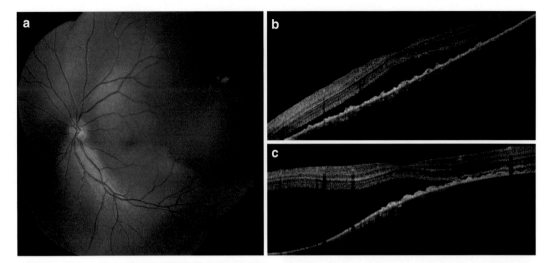

Fig. 4.28 (**a**) Shows a posterior choroidal hemangioma underlying the macula of the left eye. In the photo, there is a suggestion of subretinal fluid. OCT (**b**, horizontal; **c**, vertical cuts) shows serous retinal detachment involving the fovea, particularly inferiorly. There is atrophy of the overlying retina. The choroidal tumor itself is hyperreflective at its anterior surface and below that is hyporeflective on OCT

Acknowledgments

Dr. Carol L. Shields, MD
Dr. Jerry Shields, MD
Dr. William Benson, MD
Dr. Ehsan Rahimy, MD
Dr. Robert Sergott, MD

References

1. Wallow IH, Danis RP, Bindley C, Neider M. Cystoid macular degeneration in experimental branch retinal vein occlusion. Ophthalmology. 1998;95:1371–9.
2. Sekiruyo T, Iida T, Sakai E, et al. Fundus autofluorescence and optical coherence tomography findings in branch retinal vein occlusion. J Ophthalmol. 2012; 2012:638064.
3. Shroff D, Mehta DK, Arora R, et al. Natural history of macular status in recent-onset branch retinal vein occlusion: an optical coherence tomography study. Int Ophthalmol. 2008;28(4):261–8.
4. Spaide RF, Lee JK, Klancnik JM, Gross NE. Optical coherence tomography of branch retinal vein occlusion. Retina. 2003;23(3):343–7.
5. Kang HM, Chung EJ, Kim YM, Koh HJ. Spectral-domain optical coherence tomography (SD-OCT) patterns and response to intravitreal bevacizumab therapy in macular edema associated with branch retinal vein occlusion. Graefs Ach Clin Exp Ophthalmol. 2013;251(2):501–8.
6. Kim CS, Shin KS, Lee HJ, Jo YJ, Kim JY. Sectoral retinal nerve fiber layer thinning in branch retinal vein occlusion. Retina. 2014;34(3):525–30.
7. Castro LV, Yeung L, Castro LC, et al. Correlation between spectral domain optical coherence tomography findings and visual outcomes in central retinal vein occlusion. Clin Ophthalmol. 2001;5:299–305.
8. Martinet V, Guigui B, Glacet-Bernard A, et al. Macular edema in central retinal vein occlusion: correlation between optical coherence tomography, angiography, and visual acuity. Int Ophthalmol. 2012;32(4):369–77.
9. Rosenfeld PJ, Fung AE, Puliafito CA. Optical coherence tomography findings after an intravitreal injection of bevacizumab (Avastin) for macular edema from central retinal vein occlusion. Ophthalmic Surg Lasers Imaging. 2005;36(4):336–9.
10. Cella W, Avila M. Optical coherence tomography as a means of evaluating acute ischaemic retinopathy in branch retinal artery occlusion. Acta Ophtalmol Scand. 2007;85:799–801.
11. Karacorlu M, Ozdemir H, Arf KS. Optical coherence tomography findings in branch retinal artery occlusion. Eur J Ophthalmol. 2006;16(2):352–3.
12. Shah VA, Wallace B, Sabetes NR. Spectral domain optical coherence tomography findings of acute branch retinal artery occlusion from calcific embolus. Indian J Ophthalmol. 2010;58(6):523–4.
13. Chu YK, Hong YT, Byeon SH, Kwon OW. In vivo detection of acute ischemic damages in retinal arterial occlusion with optical coherence tomography. Retina. 2013;33(10):2110–7.
14. Falkenberry SM, Ip MS, Blodi BA, Gunther JB. Optical coherence tomography findings in central retinal artery occlusion. Ophthalmic Surg Lasers Imaging. 2006;37(6):502–5.
15. Chen SN, Hwang JF, Chen YT. Macular thickness measurements in central retinal artery occlusion by optical coherence tomography. Retina. 2011;31(4):730–7.

16. Kothari MT, Maiti A. Ophthalmic artery occlusion: a cause of unilateral visual loss following spine surgery. Indian J Ophthalmol. 2007;55(5):401–2.

17. Gaudric A, Coscas G, Bird AC. Choroidal ischemia. Am J Ophthalmol. 1982;94(4):489–98.

18. Kopsachilis N, Pefkianaki M, Marinescu A, Sivaprasad S. Giant cell arteritis presenting as choroidal infarction. Case Rep Ophthalmol Med. 2013;2013:597398.

19. Iida T, Spaide RF, Kantor J. Retinal and choroidal arterial occlusion in Wegener's granulomatosis. Am J Ophthalmol. 2002;133:151–2.

20. Viestenz A, Kuchle M. Choroidal ischaemic infarction following ocular contusion with small framed spectacles: Hutchinson-Siegrist-Neubauer- syndrome. Br J Ophthalmol. 2002;86(11):1319.

21. Contreras I, Noval S, Rebolleda G, Munoz-Negrete FJ. Follow-up of nonarteritic anterior ischemic optic neuropathy with optical coherence tomography. Ophthalmology. 2007;114(12):2338–44.

22. Tsujikawa A, Sakamoto A, Ota M, et al. Retinal structural changes associated with retinal arterial macroaneurysm examined with optical coherence tomography. Retina. 2009;29(6):782–92.

23. Lee EK, Woo SJ, Ahn A, Park KH. Morphologic characteristics of retinal arterial macroaneurysm and its regression pattern on spectral-domain optical coherence tomography. Retina. 2011;31(10):2095–101.

24. Goldenberg D, Soiberman U, Loewenstein A, Goldstein M. Heidelberg spectral-domain optical coherence tomographic findings in retinal arterial macroaneurysm. Retina. 2012;32(5):990–5.

25. Takahashi K, Kishi S. Serous macular detachment associated with retinal arterial macroaneurysm. Jpn J Ophthalmol. 2006;50(5):460–4.

26. Savar A, Vavvas D. Optical coherence tomography appearance of a retinal artery macroaneurysm. Ophthalmic Surg Lasers Imaging. 2009;40(4):403–4.

27. Horgan N, Shields CL, Mashayekhi A, Shields JA. Classification and treatment of radiation maculopathy. Curr Opin Ophthalmol. 2010;21:233–8.

28. Hong KH, Chang SD. A case of radiation retinopathy of the left eye after radiation therapy of right brain metastasis. Korean J Ophthalmol. 2009;23(2):114–7.

29. Levitz LM. The use of optical coherence tomography to determine the severity of radiation retinopathy. Ophthalmic Surg Lasers Imaging. 2005;36(5):410–1.

30. Shah SU, Shields CL, Bianciotto CG, Iturralde J, et al. Intravitreal bevacizumab at 4-month intervals for prevention of macular edema after plaque radiotherapy of uveal melanoma. Ophthalmology. 2014;121(1):269–75.

31. Purtscher O. Noch unbekannte befunde nach Schadeltrauma. Ber Dtsch Ophthalmol Ges. 1910;36: 294–301.

32. Agrawal A, McKibbon MA. Purtscher's and Purtscher-like retinopathies: a review. Surv Ophthalmol. 2006;51:129–36.

33. Agrawal A, McKibbin M. Purtscher's retinopathy: epidemiology, clinical features, and outcome. Br J Ophthalmol. 2007;91(11):1456–9.

34. Lauer AK, Klein ML, Koverik D, Palmer EA. Hemolytic uremic syndrome associated with Purtscher-like retinopathy. Arch Ophthalmol. 1998;116(8):1119–20.

35. Paunescu LA, Ko TH, Duker JS, et al. Idiopathic juxtafoveal retinal telangiectasis: New findings by ultrahigh-resolution optical coherence tomography. Ophthalmology. 2006;113:48–57.

36. Cohen SM, Cohen ML, El-Jabali F, Paulter SE. Optical coherence tomography findings in nonproliferative group 2a idiopathic juxtafoveal retinal telangiectasis. Retina. 2007;27:59–66.

37. Sanchez JG, Garcia RA, Wu L, et al. Optical coherence tomography characteristics of group 2A idiopathic parafoveal telangiectasis. Retina. 2007;27:1214–20.

38. Shukla D, Naresh KB, Kim R. Optical coherence tomography findings in valsalva retinopathy. Am J Ophthalmol. 2005;140(1):134–6.

39. Ho LY, Abdelghani WM. Valsalva retinopathy associated with the choking game. Semin Ophthalmol. 2007;22(2):63–4.

40. Zou M, Gao S, Zhang J, Zhang M. Persistent unsealed internal limiting membrane after Nd:YAG laser treatment for valsalva retinopathy. BMC Ophthalmol. 2013;13:15.

41. Park KA, Oh SY. Analysis of spectral-domain optical coherence tomography in preterm children: retinal layer thickness and choroidal thickness profiles. Invest Ophthalmol Vis Sci. 2012;53(11):7201–7.

42. Lee AC, Maldonado RS, Sarin N, et al. Macular features from spectral domain optical coherence tomography as an adjunct to indirect ophthalmoscopy in retinopathy of prematurity. Retina. 2011;31(8):1470–82.

43. Recchia FM, Recchia CC. Foveal dysplasia evident by optical coherence tomography in patients with a history of retinopathy of prematurity. Retina. 2007;27(9):1221–6.

44. Dubis AM, Subramaniam CD, Godara P, et al. Subclinical macular findings in infants screened for retinopathy of prematurity with spectral-domain optical coherence tomography. Ophthalmology. 2003;120(8):1665–71.

45. Day S, Maldonado R, Toth C. Preretinal and intraretinal exudates in familial exudative vitreoretinopathy. Retina. 2011;31(1):193–4.

46. Shimouchi A, Takahashi A, Nagaoka T, Ishibazawa A, Yoshida A. Vitreomacular interface in patients with familial vitreoretinopathy. Int Ophthalmol. 2013;33(6):711–5.

47. Otani T, Yasuda K, Aizawa N, et al. Over 10 years follow-up of Coats' disease in adulthood. Clin Ophthalmol. 2011;5:1729–32.

48. Henry CR, Berrocal AM, Hess DJ, Murray TG. Intraoperative spectral-domain optical coherence tomography in coats' disease. Ophthalmic Surg Lasers Imaging. 2012;26(43):e80–4.

49. Kamppeter B, Jonas JB. Central serous chorioreti-nopathy imaged by optical coherence tomography. Arch Ophthalmol. 2003;121(5):742–3.

50. Montero JA, Ruiz-Moreno JM. Optical coherence tomography characterization of idiopathic central serous chorioretinopathy. Br J Ophthalmol. 2005;89(5):562–4.

51. Nicholson B, Noble J, Forooghian F, Meyerle C. Central serous chorioretinopathy: update on pathophysiology and treatment. Surv Ophthalmol. 2013;58(2):103–26.

52. Yang L, Jonas JB, Wenmin W. Optical coherence tomography-assisted enhanced depth imaging of central serous chorioretinopathy. Invest Ophthalmol Vis Sci. 2013;54(7):4659–65.

53. Ojima Y, Hangai M, Sakamoto A, et al. Improved visualization of polypoidal choroidal vasculopathy lesions using spectral-domain optical coherence tomography. Retina. 2009;29(1):52–9.

54. Nagase S, Miura M, Makita S, et al. High-penetration optical coherence tomography with enhanced depth imaging of polypoidal choroidal vasculopathy. Ophthalmic Surg Lasers Imaging. 2012;9(43):e5–9.

55. Sayanagi K, Gomi F, Ikuno Y, et al. Comparison of spectral-domain and high-penetrance OCT for observing morphologic changes in age-related macular degeneration and polypoidal choroidal vasculopathy. Graefes Arch Clin Exp Ophthalmol. 2014;252(1):3–9.

56. Andrade RE, Farah ME, Costa RA, Belfort R. Optical coherence tomography findings in macular cavernous hemangioma. Acta Ophthalmol Scand. 2004;83:267–8.

57. Shields CL, Ma M, Shields JA. Review of optical coherence tomography for intraocular tumors. Curr Opin Ophthalmol. 2005;16(3):141–54.

58. Heimann H, Imor F, Damato B. Imaging of retinal and choroidal vascular tumours. Eye (Lond). 2013;27(2):208–16. doi:10.1038/eye.2012.251. Epub 2012 Nov 30.

59. Shields CL, Mashayekhi A, Luo CK, Materin MA, Shields JA. Optical coherence tomography in children: analysis of 44 eyes with intraocular tumors and simulating conditions. J Pediatr Ophthalmol Strabismus. 2004;41(6):338–44.

60. Chalam KV, Murthy RK, Gupta SK, Brar VS. Spectral domain optical coherence tomography guided photodynamic therapy for choroidal hemangioma: a case report. Cases J. 2009;2:8778–82.

Vitreomacular Adhesion/Traction Syndromes

5

David A. Salz

Abstract

Vitreomacular adhesion and traction syndromes are diseases involving pathologic interaction of the vitreoretinal interface. These diseases have been greater delineated with the advent of spectral domain OCT, which has allowed for precise imaging leading to greater description and understanding of the various disease processes. This chapter demonstrates via case examples a variety of vitreomacular and vitreoretinal syndromes, their clinical presentations, and OCT characteristics.

Keywords

Vitreomacular traction • Vitreomacular adhesion • Epiretinal membrane • Vitreopapillary traction • Macular hole • Lamellar hole

Vitreomacular Adhesion and Traction

Vitreomacular adhesion is classically defined as when the posterior hyaloid face does not completely separate from the retina, but remains adhered to the macula. There are typically no symptoms with vitreomacular adhesion as the retina is not distorted and is anatomically normal. However, if the attachment persists, and begins pulling at the retina, it can begin to pull at the retina, causing symptoms of distortion or loss of vision, and is then called vitreomacular traction. Vitreomacular traction is defined as an acquired retinal disease where there is partial separation of the posterior hyaloid face with an area of persistent attachment to the macula causing anatomic distortion of the fovea [1]. Vitreomacular traction typically occurs in patients who are 50 or older, which is the same age as patients who are likely to have a posterior vitreous detachment.

Vitreomacular traction can be hard to see discretely on fundoscopic exam. Patients often complain of distortion or decreased vision. Clinically, one can sometimes see a blunted reflex or occasionally some foveal edema or striae, but often this condition is hard to detect.

D.A. Salz, MD
Department of Ophthalmology, Wills Eye Hospital, Philadelphia, PA, USA
e-mail: dasalz@gmail.com

© Springer International Publishing Switzerland 2016
A. Girach, R.C. Sergott (eds.), *Optical Coherence Tomography*,
DOI 10.1007/978-3-319-24817-2_5

69

OCT has allowed for much more precise imaging of the vitreoretinal interface and led to much better comprehension of the pathophysiologic as well as diagnosis of the vitreomacular adhesion and traction syndrome [2].

In December 2013, the International Vitreomacular Traction Study (IVTS) Group published in *Ophthalmology* a new anatomic classification system for vitreomacular adhesion, traction, and macular hole relying solely on OCT features. Their definition of vitreomacular adhesion is perifoveal separation with remaining vitreomacular attachment and unperturbed foveal morphologic features. Vitreomacular traction is characterized by anomalous posterior vitreous detachment accompanied by anatomic distortion of the fovea, which may include pseudocysts, macular schisis, cystoid macular edema, and subretinal fluid. Vitreomacular traction can also be subdivided by the diameter of vitreous attach-

ment to the macular surface. Using OCT measurement parameters, an attachment of 1500 μm or less is classified as focal, with larger than 1500 μm attachments classified as broad [3].

Case 1

A 54-year-old female presents with noting slight blurring of her left eye over the past 2 weeks. She denies any new flashes or floaters. Past medical history is significant for cholecystectomy 10 years prior. Snellen visual acuity was 20/20 OD and 20/30 OS. Dilated fundoscopic examination revealed a blunted foveal reflex in the left eye. An OCT was obtained as shown in Figs. 5.1 and 5.2.

The decision was made to observe given the mild vision loss. The condition fortunately resolved on its own with complete release of the vitreous traction and resolution of the vision to 20/20.

Fig. 5.1 An area of vitreomacular traction is present creating distortion of the fovea. Note the areas of adhesion of the posterior hyaloid face causing focal elevation of the retina with intraretinal edema

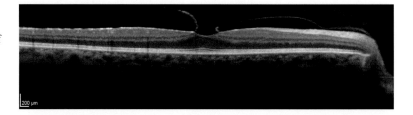

Fig. 5.2 The asymptomatic eye. Note the area of vitreomacular adhesion that is present but not causing any pathologic changes. It is not uncommon to see some element of vitreomacular interface pathology in both eyes, as it is believed the vitreoretinal interface interaction is abnormal in both eyes

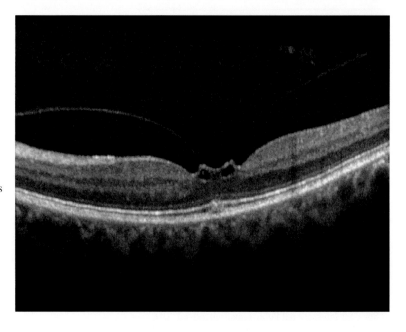

Case 2

A 63-year-old male presents with decreased vision in the left eye for 2 months, that has continued to progress. He reports distortion of his vision as well. His past medical history is significant for hypertension, hyperlipidemia, and skin melanoma status post complete resection. Snellen visual acuity was 20/25 OD and 20/80 OS. Dilated fundoscopic examination was notable for an abnormal foveal reflex in the left eye with a few fine retinal striae. An OCT was done as shown in Fig. 5.3.

Given the worsening vision and severe traction, the patient underwent a pars plana vitrectomy with ultimate improvement of the vision to 20/25 and anatomic restoration of the foveal depression and resolution of the macular edema.

With the recent FDA approval of ocriplasmin in 2013, enzymatic vitreous adhesion lysis offers another potential intervention that could be beneficial for this syndrome. In the MIVI-TRUST trials, a complete posterior vitreous detachment was pharmacologically induced in 13.4 % of patients at 28 days after injection of ocriplasmin ($P<0.001$) [4]. Intervention to cause release of the traction can lead to restoration of the anatomy, as well as functional vision improvement, while avoiding a surgical procedure.

Surgical intervention with pars plana vitrectomy has been shown to be effective for vitreomacular traction. A large retrospective done by Witkin et al. on patients with vitreomacular traction syndrome showed an improvement in both mean visual acuity from 20/122 preoperatively to 20/68 postoperatively. There was also significant improvement in mean fovea thickness, with a decrease from 404 to 251 μm after surgery [5].

Lamellar Holes

The term lamellar macular hole was first coined by Gass in 1975 [6]. Lamellar holes are partial thickness retinal holes in the fovea with intact photoreceptors. OCT has helped redefine these lesions, typically seen on fundoscopic exam as a reddish foveal lesion. Because lamellar holes can sometimes appear to be a full-thickness hole on examination, it is also sometimes called a pseudohole. Lamellar holes are thought to be created by a similar pathogenesis to macular holes and vitreomacular traction. A large number of patients with lamellar holes also have epiretinal membranes. Patients typically have relatively preserved vision.

The diagnosis of lamellar macular holes has been greatly aided by the advent of OCT. In a study done by Haouchine et al., only 28 % of lamellar holes were diagnosed on fundus examination as compared with OCT [7]. OCT typically shows preserved outer retinal layers with intact photoreceptors but an absence or avulsion of the inner layers. According to a recent classification by Witkin et al., there are four OCT criteria needed for the diagnosis of a lamellar macular hole. These are an irregular foveal contour, a break in the inner fovea, separation of the inner from outer foveal retinal layers, and absence of a full-thickness foveal defect with intact photoreceptors [8].

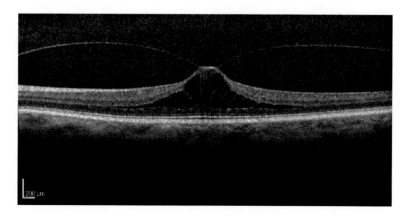

Fig. 5.3 A focal area of vitreomacular traction is present in the fovea, causing complete loss of the foveal depression. There are large discrete areas of cystic intraretinal edema

Case 1

A 67-year-old female was referred for a retinal exam status post cataract extraction in her left eye. She had a history of cataract surgery in both eyes with no complications. The patient noted the vision did not seem quite as crisp in the left eye, but was not that bad. She reported no other symptoms. Past medical history was significant for diabetes mellitus type II, coronary artery disease, and degenerative joint disease. Her corrected Snellen visual acuity was 20/40 OD and 20/25 OS. Pupils were equal and reactive in both eyes with no afferent pupillary defect. Fundus examination revealed normal foveal contour in the right eye and an irregular reddish foveal lesion in the left eye. OCT was obtained and is shown below in Fig. 5.4.

Case 2

A 77-year-old male presents with complaints of visual distortion in his left eye. He denies any trauma or other ocular complaints. He has a history of blepharitis in both eyes as well as successful cataract surgery 10 years prior. His past medical history is significant for colon cancer and hypertension. Snellen visual acuity was 20/20 in the right eye and 20/40 in the left eye. Examination revealed well-centered posterior chamber intraocular lenses in both eyes, as well as an irregular foveal reflex in the left eye with a few striae temporal to the fovea. OCT was done which is shown in Fig. 5.5.

In both of these cases, the decision was made to observe the patient. Because lamellar holes are not full thickness, vision is generally relatively preserved, and the patient is often asymptomatic, although certainly not always. Many prospective studies have shown various efficacies of a pars plana vitrectomy surgical approach for intervention, with some showing minimal improvement, and thus surgery should be exercised with caution.

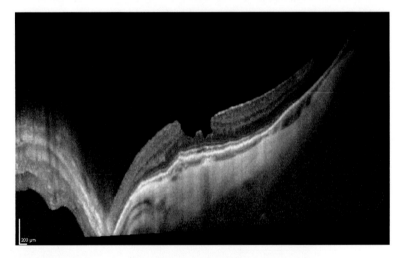

Fig. 5.4 Note the abnormality of the foveal depression as well as the loss of the inner retinal layers. Also note that the outer photoreceptor layers are intact, making this a lamellar hole as opposed to a full-thickness macular hole

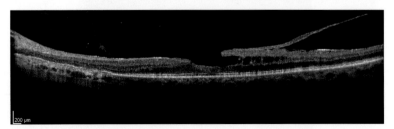

Fig. 5.5 Note the area of vitreomacular adhesion temporal to the fovea pulling the retina, causing avulsion of the inner retinal layers. The photoreceptors are still intact and the IS/OS junction is well preserved, which is why the patient still has good vision. Also, an epiretinal membrane is present; note the hyperreflective and slightly irregular surface of the retina nasally

Macular Holes

A macular hole is defined as a retinal hole typically involving the fovea. The etiology is most commonly idiopathic, although myopia, age, trauma, female sex, and ocular inflammation are all risk factors. It has been hypothesized that macular holes are caused by tangential traction of the posterior hyaloid face on the parafoveal region. Symptoms included decreased vision, metamorphopsia, or a central scotoma [9].

Classically, macular holes were divided by fundus appearance. There are four stages described by the Gass Classification. Stage 1 macular holes are an impending hole with loss of foveal depression. Stage 1A is a foveolar detachment characterized by a loss of the foveal contour and a yellow spot (from lipofuscin). A stage 1B is a foveal detachment characterized by a yellow-colored ring. Stage 2 macular holes are defined as a full-thickness central or paracentral break less than 400 μm in size, with an associated cuff of subretinal fluid. Stage 3 macular holes are greater than 400 μm in size with detachment of the posterior hyaloid face from the macula. Stage 4 macular holes are the same as stage 3 except there is a complete posterior vitreous detachment [10, 11].

The IVTS recently reclassified a full-thickness macular hole to be defined as a full-thickness foveal lesion with interruption of all retinal layers from the internal limiting membrane to the retinal pigment epithelium. Macular holes are defined as primary if caused by vitreous traction and secondary if from any other cause. Subclassifications are determined by the size of the hole as well as the presence or absence of vitreomacular traction. The size classification is determined by the horizontal linear width across the hole at the narrowest point and has three categories: small (<250 μm), medium (>250 μm but <400 μm), and large (>400 μm) [3].

Case 1

A 61-year-old white female reported decreasing vision in her right eye for 3 years and 2 months of decreased vision in her left eye. Snellen visual acuity was 20/400 OD and 20/80 OS. A relative afferent pupillary defect was observed in the right eye, and color plates were 0/9 in her right eye and 9/9 in her left eye. Humphrey 24–2 visual fields showed inferior and superior arcuate defects with paracentral defects in the right eye and a normal visual field in the left eye.

Dilated fundoscopic examination revealed a hyperpigmented lesion of the retinal pigment epithelium [RPE] in the right eye surrounding a dysplastic optic nerve with a dense tractional band of fibrosis extending from the lesion into the vitreous, as well as macular edema (Fig. 5.6). The left eye showed a full-thickness macular hole (Fig. 5.7). SD-OCT demonstrated marked peripapillary retinal disk elevation temporally in the right eye, with elevation of the retinal nerve fiber layer in all four quadrants. The OCT also confirmed edema in the outer nuclear area of the macula (Figs. 5.8 and 5.9). The OCT of the left eye confirmed the macular hole (Fig. 5.10). A clinical diagnosis of combined hamartoma of the sensory retina and retinal pigment epithelium was made. The patient first underwent vitrectomy in the left eye for the macular hole with membrane peel and C_3F_8 gas, followed by cataract extraction. Two months later, vitrectomy was performed in the right eye. Final visual acuity was 20/200 OD with resolution of the vitreopapillary traction and 20/25 OS.

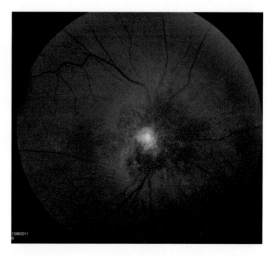

Fig. 5.6 Congenital peripapillary hamartoma of the retinal pigment epithelium of the right eye in association with dysplasia of the optic nerve

Case 2

A 73-year-old white female presents with decreased vision in her left eye for 2 weeks. She cannot describe when her visual acuity decreased, but she realized it while reading a newspaper and covered each eye. Her past medical history is significant for hypertension, hypothyroidism, and osteoporosis. Snellen visual acuity is 20/30 OD and 20/100 OS. Dilated fun-

doscopic exam is notable for a full-thickness macular hole in the left eye. Watzke–Allen test is performed, which consists of bringing a slit beam over the macula. If the patient states it disappears, then it confirms that a full-thickness hole is present. An OCT was done and is shown in Fig. 5.11.

The patient underwent pars plana vitrectomy with internal limiting membrane peel with complete closure of the hole and improvement in vision to 20/40.

Epiretinal Membranes

Epiretinal membranes are defined as cellular proliferation along the internal limiting membrane and retinal surface causing a semitransparent fibrocellular membrane. If the membrane contracts, the retinal surface can become wrinkled, which is called macular pucker or cellophane retinopathy. Risk factors for an epiretinal membrane include age, prior retinal surgery, intraocular inflammation, posterior vitreous detachment, intraocular tumors, and trauma. Epiretinal membranes can also be idiopathic. It is thought that a posterior vitreous detachment may induce some

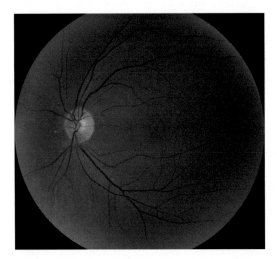

Fig. 5.7 Normal appearance of the optic disk with full-thickness macular hole of the left eye. Note the central retinal pigment epithelial changes in the hole and the surrounding cuff of subretinal fluid around the hole

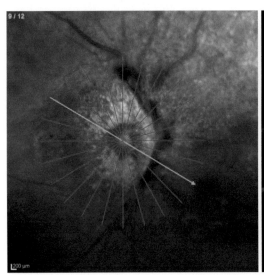
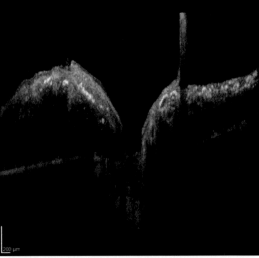

Fig. 5.8 SD-OCT of the right optic nerve demonstrating peripapillary traction with elevation of the neurosensory retina and underlying subretinal fluid

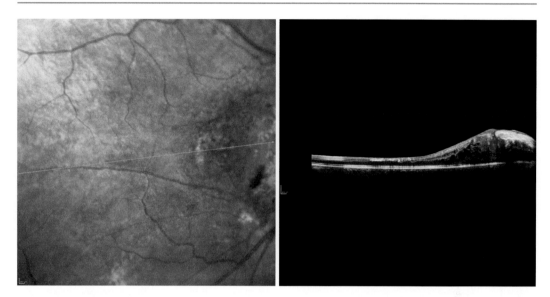

Fig. 5.9 Longitudinal SD-OCT of right eye demonstrating extension of the subretinal fluid and intraretinal cystoid edema beyond the immediately adjacent peripapillary area

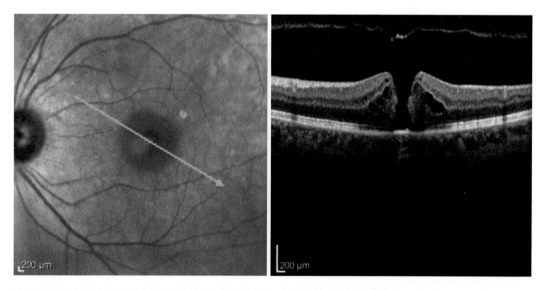

Fig. 5.10 Full-thickness macular hole of the left eye with surrounding cystoid macular edema. Note the complete hole, with no IS/OS junction present and complete retinal tissue loss in the fovea. There is a full posterior vitreous detachment that can be seen overlying the retina. This is a stage 4 full-thickness macular hole

residual posterior vitreous that is left on the macula to proliferate or disrupt the internal limiting membrane, causing metaplasia to glial cells and formation of an epiretinal membrane [1]. Mild epiretinal membranes do not cause symptoms, but as the membrane grows and contracts, visual symptoms include decreased vision, macropsia or micropsia, metamorphopsia, and monocular diplopia.

Clinically, epiretinal membranes appear as a translucent, glistening membrane in the macula. OCT is very useful for delineating and diagnosing epiretinal membranes. OCT features include an extra layer on the inner part of the retina which appears as a hyperreflective band which can have associated retinal thickening, macular edema, and loss of the normal retinal contour. Epiretinal membranes cause also cause macular pseudoholes to form, which appear clinically to be full-thickness holes, but OCT reveals a partial thickness hole with preservation of the outer retinal layers (see lamellar hole) [9]. This can sometimes be distinguished clinically using the Watzke-Allen test.

Treatment of epiretinal membranes consists of either observation or pars plana vitrectomy with membrane peel. Given the inherent risks, surgery is typically limited to patients with 20/50 vision or worse or with severe refractory symptoms.

Case 1

A 57-year-old male presents with complaints of swirling blurry vision in his left eye for 3 months. He has a history of floaters in both eyes for about

5 years. He has a history of non-insulin-dependent diabetes mellitus and a remote history of non-Hodgkin's lymphoma. Snellen visual acuity is 20/20 OD and 20/30 OS. Amsler grid reveals distortion of the central vision in the left eye. Pupils are equal and reactive with no afferent pupillary defect. Dilated fundoscopic examination reveals an epiretinal membrane in the left eye with blunting of the foveal reflex. OCT is obtained which is shown in Fig. 5.12.

Optic Disk/Peripapillary Traction Syndromes

Vitreous–papillary and peripapillary traction has been described in the literature occurring from various causes, most commonly in association with diabetic retinopathy [12]. Vitreous–papillary and peripapillary traction is characterized by

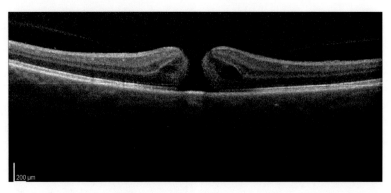

Fig. 5.11 Stage 2 macular hole. There is still vitreous attached to the macula at the edge of the fovea on both sides. Also, note the intraretinal edema and complete loss of all retinal layers centrally. The patient underwent pars plana vitrectomy with internal limiting membrane peel with complete closure of the hole and improvement in vision to 20/40

Fig. 5.12 Note the hyperreflective band on the surface of the retina causing loss of the foveal depression and retinal thickening. Given the patient's good visual acuity, the decision was made to observe with the plan to intervene if the symptoms or the vision became worse

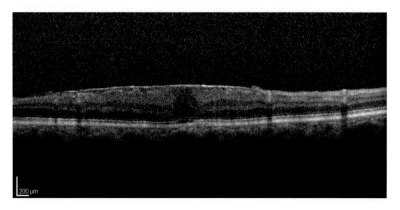

a fibrocellular membrane or incomplete vitreous detachment exerting force on the optic disk and the surrounding tissue [13, 14].

While vitreomacular adhesion has been well described in the literature, there has been less focus on vitreous–papillary adhesion. This interface is difficult to evaluate clinically. In earlier studies, such as Katz and Hoyt in 2005, B-scan ultrasonography was used to determine if a posterior vitreous detachment or adhesion of vitreous to the optic nerve was present [15]. Spectral–domain optical coherence tomography images the vitreous–papillary interface with greater resolution and with microscopic, precise detail, enabling the accurate clinical diagnosis of vitreous–optic disk–peripapillary retinal traction syndromes.

Case 1

A 43-year-old male truck driver presented for consultation with complaints of hazy vision in the right eye for several years. Snellen visual acuity was 20/20 OD and 20/25 OS. A relative afferent pupillary defect was observed in his right eye, and color plates were 4/9 OD and 9/9 OS. Visual fields found a superior and inferior nerve fiber layer defect in the right eye and some scattered areas of decreased sensitivity in the left eye. Anterior segment examination was white and quiet in both eyes.

Dilated fundoscopic examination showed diffuse optic nerve pallor in the right eye with peripapillary chorioretinal and retinal pigment atrophy inferiorly (Fig. 5.13). Subtle yellowish deposits were present superiorly, nasally, and temporally to the optic disk suggesting a possible prior subclinical inflammatory optic neuropathy. Both eyes had foveal RPE mottling. OCT scan showed a thick band of vitreous elevating the optic disk with decreased peripapillary retinal nerve fiber layer thickness in all quadrants except in the papillomacular bundle, which was thickened (Figs. 5.14 and 5.15). The left eye was within normal limits. The patient underwent vitrectomy, which was complicated by significant postoperative inflammation and concern for endophthalmitis. He underwent a vitreous tap

and intravitreal injection of antibiotics. The vitreous sample grew *Propionibacterium acnes*. Vision recovered to 20/20 at 1-year follow-up, with stabilization of the optic neuropathy.

Case 2

A 58-year-old female with a history of sarcoidosis and chronic optic disk swelling presented with declining vision from 20/20 in her right eye to 20/60 over 3 years. She complained of curved vision on the right side of her vision in her right eye. Slit-lamp examination was notable for a moderate vitreous cellular reaction in the right eye and mild nuclear sclerosis in both eyes. Visual field was notable for central and paracentral scotomas. MRI scanning did not show any enhancement of the optic nerves, chiasm, posterior afferent visual system, or the meninges.

Fundoscopic exam revealed RPE depigmentation nasal and inferior to the optic nerve with fibrous tissue on the optic nerve head with striae extending out, as well as an epiretinal membrane (Fig. 5.16). The left eye was normal. OCT confirmed the optic nerve traction and epiretinal membrane in the right

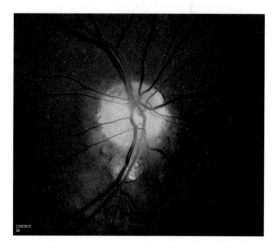

Fig. 5.13 Diffuse pallor of the optic disk of the right eye of patient 2 with surrounding peripapillary hypo- and hyperpigmentation. Subtle punctate yellowish areas are seen superiorly, nasally, and temporally, approximately one disk diameter away from the margin of the optic nerve. These areas may be consistent with prior exudate, suggesting a possible prior inflammatory optic neuropathy with disk edema

Fig. 5.14 SD-OCT showing thick traction bands attached to the nasal temporal margins of the optic disk of patient 2

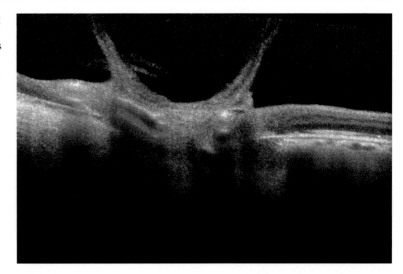

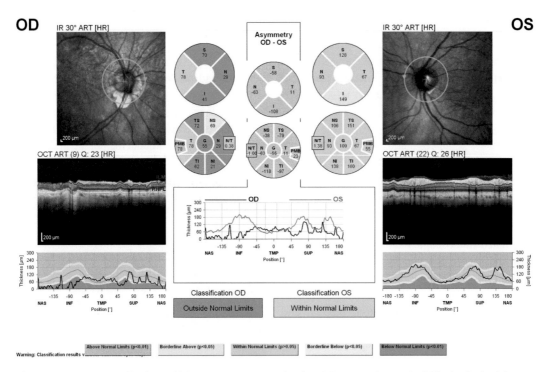

Fig. 5.15 Retinal nerve fiber layer thickness measurements of patient 2 demonstrating marked thinning in the right eye. Left eye is normal

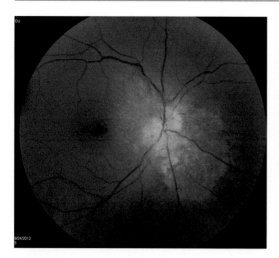

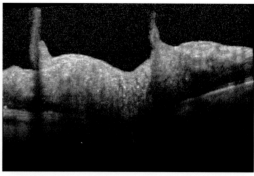

Fig. 5.17 Dense vitreopapillary traction bands of patient 3 with chronic optic disk edema and increased hyporeflectivity in the subretinal, peripapillary space

Fig. 5.16 Chronic retinal nerve fiber layer edema temporally with retinal fold extending superiorly and inferiorly as well as to the macula of patient 3 in association with atrophy of the retinal pigment epithelium inferiorly and nasally

eye (Fig. 5.17). The patient underwent vitrectomy, with improvement of the vision to 20/20. The visual field also improved, with mean deviation decreasing from −6.56 to −4.09 and decreased size and density of her scotomas.

References

1. Fineman MS, Ho AC, Rapuano CJ, Brown GC. Color atlas and synopsis of clinical ophthalmology. Wills Eye Institute atlas series: retina. Philadelphia: Lippincott Williams & Wilkins; 2012.
2. Bottos JM, Elizalde J, Rodrigues EB, Maia M. Current concepts in vitreomacular traction syndrome. Curr Opin Ophthalmol. 2012;23:195–201.
3. Duker JS, Kaiser PK, Binder S, de Smet MD, Gaudric A, Reichel E, et al. The International Viteromacular Traction Study Group classification of viteromacular adhesion, traction, and macular hole. Ophthalmology. 2013;120:2611–9.
4. Stalmans P, Benz MS, Gandorfer A, Kampik A, Girach A, Pakola S, Haller JA, MIVI-TRUST Study Group. Enzymatic vitreolysis with ocriplasmin for vitreomacular traction and macular holes. N Engl J Med. 2012;367:606–15.
5. Witkin AJ, Patron ME, Castro LC, Reichel E, Rogers AH, Baumal CR, Duker JS. Anatomic and visual outcomes of vitrectomy for vitreomacular trac-
   tion syndrome. Ophthalmic Surg Lasers Imaging. 2010;41:425–31.
6. Gass JD. Lamellar macular hole: a complication of cystoid macular edema after cataract extraction: a clinicopathologic case report. Trans Am Ophthalmol Soc. 1975;73:230–50.
7. Haouchine B, Massin P, Tadayoni R, Erginay A, Gaudric A. Diagnosis of macular pseudoholes and lamellar macular holes by optical coherence tomography. Am J Ophthalmol. 2004;138:732–9.
8. Witkin A, Ko TH, Fujimoto JG, Schuman JS, Baumal CR, Rogers AH, et al. Redefining lamellar holes and the vitreomacular interface: ultrahigh resolution optical coherence tomography study. Ophthalmology. 2006;113:388–97.
9. Steel DW, Lotery AJ. Idiopathic vitreomacular traction and macular hole: a comprehensive review of pathophysiology, diagnosis, and treatment. Eye. 2013;27:S1–21.
10. Gass JD. Reappraisal of biomicroscopic classification of stages of development of a macular hole. Am J Ophthalmol. 1995;119:752–9.
11. Gass JD. Idiopathic senile macular hole: its early stages and pathogenesis. Arch Ophthalmol. 1988;106:629–39.
12. Kroll P, Wiegand W, Schmidt J. Vitreopapillary traction in proliferative diabetic vitreoretinopathy. Br J Ophthalmol. 1999;83:261–4.
13. Houle E, Miller NR. Bilateral vitreopapillary traction demonstrated by optical coherence tomography mistaken for papilledema. Case Rep Ophthalmol Med. 2012;2012:682659.
14. Johnson MW. Posterior vitreous detachment: evolution and complications of its early stages. Am J Ophthalmol. 2010;149:371–82.
15. Katz B, Hoyt WF. Gaze evoked amaurosis from vitreopapillary traction. Am J Ophthalmol. 2005;139:631–7.

Toxic and Nutritional Conditions

6

David H. Perlmutter

Abstract

Medication and nutritional exposures can cause peripapillary retinal nerve fiber layer changes. Cases of linezolid-induced optic neuropathy, toxic optic neuropathy secondary to paclitaxel, neuroferritinopathy, tobacco alcohol amblyopia, and thiamine deficiency are discussed.

Keywords

Linezolid • Paclitaxel • Carboplatin • Neuroferritinopathy • Tobacco alcohol amblyopia • Thiamine deficiency

Medication and nutritional exposures can cause peripapillary retinal nerve fiber layer changes. Cases of linezolid-induced optic neuropathy, toxic optic neuropathy secondary to paclitaxel, neuroferritinopathy, tobacco alcohol amblyopia, and thiamine deficiency are discussed.

Case 1

A 55-year-old male with a history of diabetes mellitus type 2, hypertension, and peripheral vascular disease status post left lower extremity bypass and status post right below the knee amputation presented with 6 weeks of worsening vision in both eyes. He describes a shadow in front of both eyes, like a "gray leaf" above the horizontal meridian. He also describes difficulty seeing red lights at nighttime, and he reports that green lights fade into other lights into the nighttime. He compensates for this by moving his eyes eccentrically to focus his vision. He previously underwent a computed tomography scan of the brain, which was negative for acute changes, as well as carotid Doppler ultrasounds, which demonstrated less than 50 % stenosis bilaterally.

He is on numerous medications, including metronidazole, nortriptyline, linezolid, gabapentin, metformin, glipizide, ramipril, pantoprazole, and warfarin.

On examination, his vision was 20/100 in the right eye and 20/50 in the left eye, without improvement on pinhole. Color plates were 1 of 11 on the right and 4 of 11 on the left. There was

D.H. Perlmutter, MD
Department of Ophthalmology, Wills Eye Hospital,
Philadelphia, PA, USA
e-mail: dhperlmutter@gmail.com

© Springer International Publishing Switzerland 2016
A. Girach, R.C. Sergott (eds.), *Optical Coherence Tomography*,
DOI 10.1007/978-3-319-24817-2_6

8

no relative afferent pupillary defect. The remainder of the anterior segment and posterior segment exam were unremarkable.

His Humphrey visual field showed bilateral central scotomas (Fig. 6.1a, b). Brain MRI with and without contrast was normal. Laboratory workup results for vitamin B12, folate, methyl-malonic acid, Lyme, ANA, CRP, ESR, RPR, ACE, and CBC were all within normal limits.

His OCT showed normal-appearing retina horizontal scans, but a mild increase in the retinal nerve fiber layer thickness in both eyes (Figs. 6.2 and 6.3).

The OCT changes resolved with discontinuation of the linezolid. The central scotomas

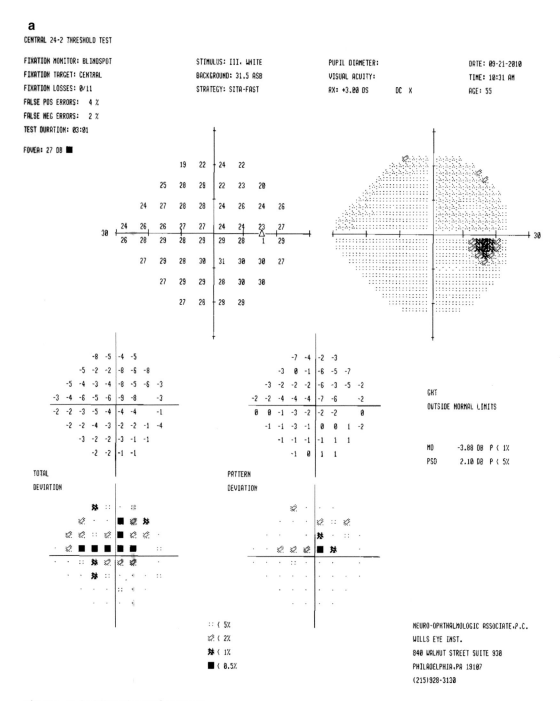

Fig. 6.1 (**a**, **b**) Bilateral central scotomas

b

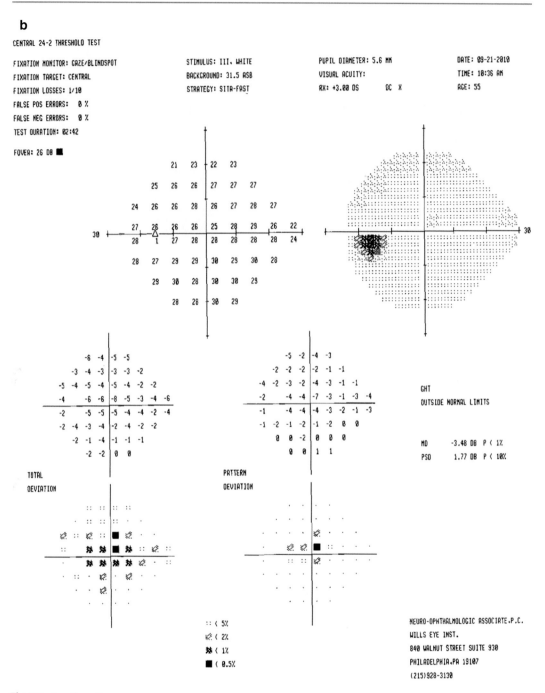

Fig. 6.1 (continued)

improved as well. On a 3-week follow-up visit, vision was 20/50 in the right eye and 20/40 in the left eye. Color plates were 8 of 15 on the right and 12 of 15 on the left. The remainder of the anterior segment exam was within normal limits, and posterior exam was notable for trace optic nerve pallor in both eyes. At 4 months of follow-up, the vision improved to 20/25 in the right eye and 20/30 in the left eye. Color vision was full in both eyes, and the anterior and posterior segment exams were notable for trace optic pallor in both eyes.

The patient was diagnosed with linezolid-induced optic neuropathy. Linezolid is an

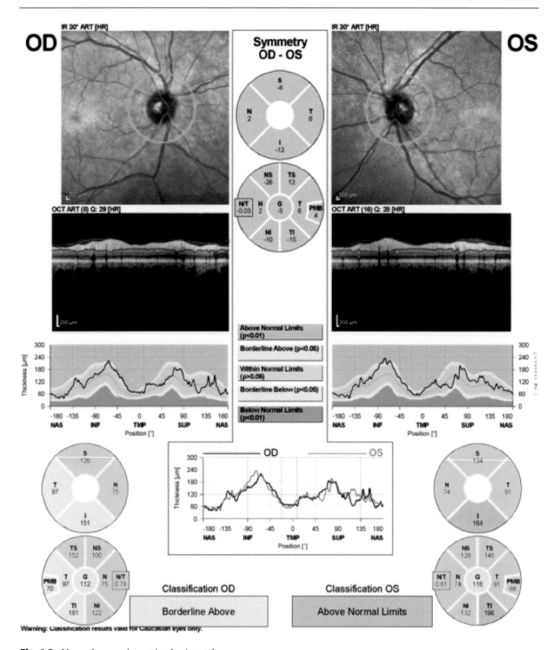

Fig. 6.2 Normal-appearing retina horizontal scans

oxazolidinone antimicrobial. It inhibits bacterial protein synthesis at the early translational stage [1]. Documented cases of optic neuropathy have been reported in patients being treated with conditions ranging from methicillin-resistant *Staphylococcus aureus* (MRSA) infection to multidrug-resistant tuberculosis (MDR TB) infection [2, 3]. Duration of therapy has been

reported ranging from 16 days to many months [4, 5]. Symptoms can include enlarged blind spot and central scotoma, which usually improve with discontinuation of the medication [4]. Although the rate of this adverse effect is not well known, a review of 30 patients treated in California for MDR TB documented one instance of optic neuropathy [6].

OD, IR 30° ART + OCT 30° ART (100) Q: 33 [HR]

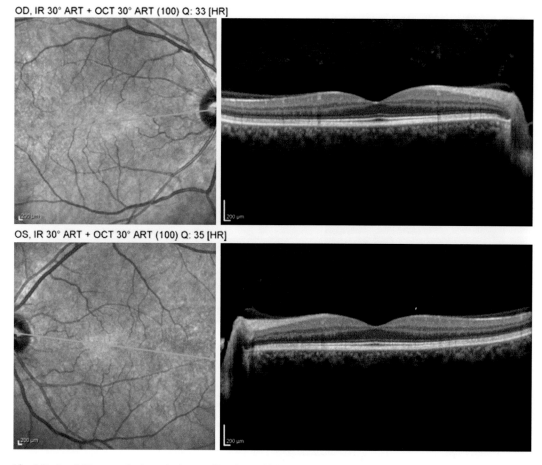

OS, IR 30° ART + OCT 30° ART (100) Q: 35 [HR]

Fig. 6.3 A mild increase in the retinal nerve fiber layer thickness in both eyes

Case 2

A 55-year-old female with a history of breast cancer status post resection and ovarian cancer presented with colorful circles and visual phenomenon while receiving carboplatin and paclitaxel chemotherapy for her breast cancer. She was on chemotherapy for 6 months, completing her course 2 months prior to this presentation. Those phenomena resolved after cessation of chemotherapy, but she notes a residual visual field defect in both eyes.

Medications include Nexium, Creon, simvastatin, alprazolam, lidocaine, Ambien, ibuprofen, and Lexapro.

Her exam showed 20/20 vision in both eyes, with full color vision in both eyes as well. There was no afferent pupillary defect. Anterior and posterior segment examinations were remarkable only for nasal elevation of her optic nerves, more on the right than on the left.

Humphrey visual field showed temporal field changes in the left eye greater than the right eye.

An MRI of the orbits and brain with and without contrast showed no mass lesions and no pituitary abnormalities.

OCT showed increased peripapillary retinal nerve fiber layer thickness inferiorly in both eyes with normal macular contour bilaterally (Figs. 6.4 and 6.5). Vitreomacular/vitreopapillary adhesion was present without traction. The patient and oncologist were notified that the optic nerve edema and visual field deficit could be secondary to either carboplatin, paclitaxel, or a combination of the two medications. The medications were discontinued.

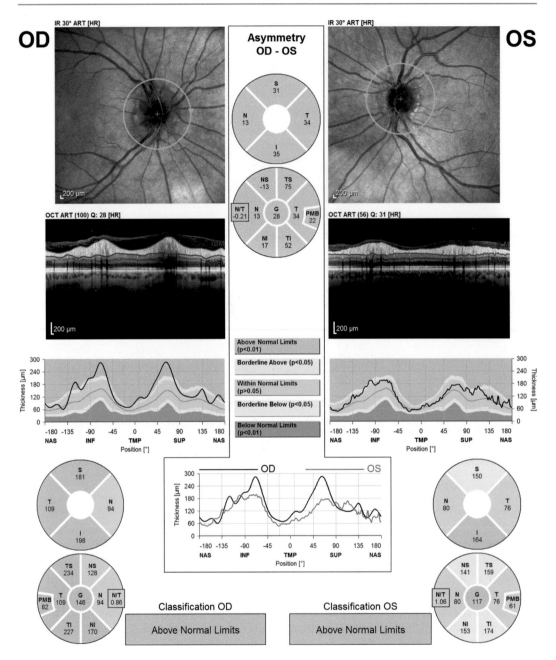

Fig. 6.4 OCT showed increased peripapillary retinal nerve fiber layer thickness inferiorly in both eyes with normal macular contour bilaterally

At 2 months of follow-up, there was improvement in the peripapillary retinal nerve fiber layer thickness in both eyes. The patient was diagnosed with a toxic optic neuropathy secondary to paclitaxel use.

Paclitaxel is a chemotherapeutic medication in the taxane class of medicines [7]. It works by stabilizing microtubules to prevent disassembly during mitosis and therefore inhibits cell turnover. Early reports described ocular

OD, IR 30° ART + OCT 30° (8.8 mm) ART (62) Q: 39 [HR]

OS, IR 30° ART + OCT 30° (8.6 mm) ART (80) Q: 38 [HR]

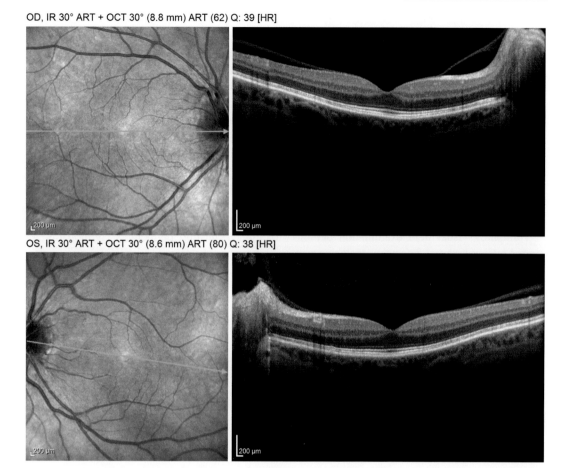

Fig. 6.5 OCT showed increased peripapillary retinal nerve fiber layer thickness inferiorly in both eyes with normal macular contour bilaterally

side effects and toxicity of the medication, including scintillating scotomas, during infusion of the medication, which resolved with completion of the infusion [8]. One group of authors looked at visual evoked potentials (VEP), oscillatory potentials (OP), and white flash electroretinograms (ERG) before and after paclitaxel treatment. Visual symptoms were not well correlated with VEP or ERG findings, but they were correlated with mild attenuation of the OP [9].

Carboplatin is a chemotherapeutic medication in the platinum-based class of compounds. It has been associated with optic nerve edema [10] and both reversible and permanent optic neuropathy. Cisplatin, a stronger platinum-based medication,

has been reported to cause optic nerve changes. Patients who received combination treatment with cisplatin, which prevents cell mitosis by cross-linking DNA, and paclitaxel had significantly decreased RNFL measurements and frequency-doubling technology perimetry values after treatment compared with their baseline results [11].

Case 3

A 40-year-old male with a history of neuroferritinopathy presented with generalized blurring of the vision in both eyes over 3 weeks. He receives regular iron chelation treatments for neuroferritinopathy and reports some visual improvement following treatments.

He smokes three quarters of a pack of cigarettes daily and consumes one alcoholic beverage weekly.

On exam, visual acuity was 20/40 in the right eye and 20/60 in the left eye. Color vision was limited to the test plate only in both eyes. Pupils were sluggish in both eyes without relative afferent pupillary defect or anisometropia. There was bilateral upgaze restriction of about 50 % in each eye. Anterior segment examination was unremarkable, and posterior segment examination was significant for optic nerve pallor in both eyes.

Humphrey visual field examination demonstrated bilateral central defects, as well as a possible left homonymous pattern.

OCT of both eyes showed epiretinal membrane changes and discontinuity of the junction of the outer and inner retinal. The left eye had additional inner retinal cystic spaces (Fig. 6.6). On multicolor imaging, there is a loss of both superficial and deep retinal reflectivity (Fig. 6.7a–d). Globally, RNFL thinning was present in both eyes (Fig. 6.8).

Iron has an essential role in retinal and optic nerve physiology. Abnormalities in iron levels, or treatment for elevated levels, can cause optic nerve or retinal abnormalities. There are multiple reports of iron chelation therapy with deferoxamine causing pigmentary retinopathy in adults and children [12, 13]. In one series, only 1.2 % of patients receiving therapy with

OD, IR 30° ART + OCT 30° (8.6 mm) ART (66) Q: 39 [HR]

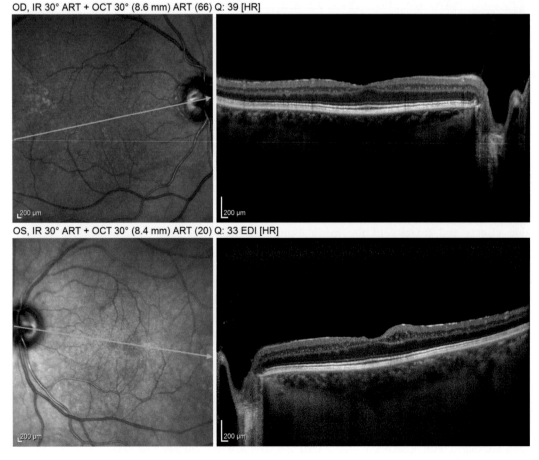

OS, IR 30° ART + OCT 30° (8.4 mm) ART (20) Q: 33 EDI [HR]

Fig. 6.6 The left eye had additional inner retinal cystic spaces

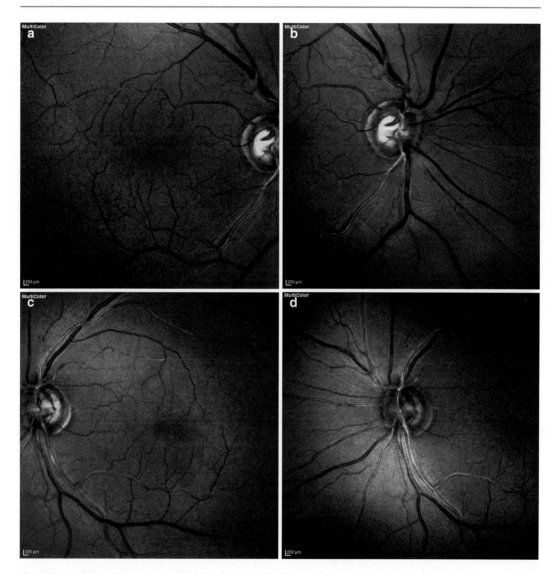

Fig. 6.7 (a–d) On multicolor imaging, there is a loss of both superficial and deep retinal reflectivity

deferoxamine had abnormalities on evaluation by an ophthalmologist. Higher levels of iron, in contrast, have been identified histopathologically in eyes with age-related macular degeneration, and it is surmised that iron may have a role in the pathogenesis of AMD through free-radical production [14, 15]. Iron is actively transported into the retina across the blood-retinal barrier, which is maintained independently by the retinal vasculature and the retinal pigment epithelium. Histopathology in iron-overload syndromes such as hemochromatosis has shown iron deposits in the peripapillary retinal pigment epithelium, as well as drusen deposition containing iron [16].

Case 4

A 58-year-old male with a recent history of a 1-month hospital admission for urosepsis presented with slowly decreasing vision in both eyes that is worse on the left than the right. He also reported recent unintentional weight loss

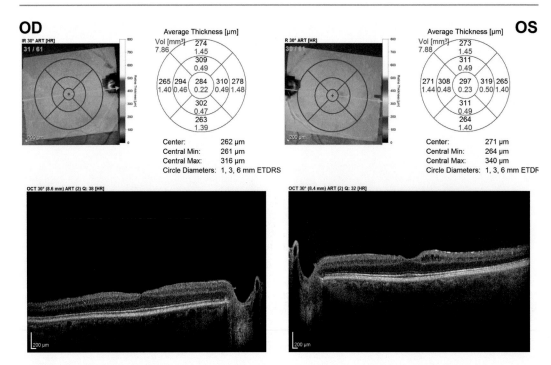

Fig. 6.8 Globally, RNFL thinning was present in both eyes

and fatigue, with decrease oral intake since his hospitalization. He smoked a quarter pack of cigarettes per day for 47 years and denied alcohol or drug use.

His medications included vitamin B12 injections, Celexa, and a multivitamin

On exam, visual acuity was 20/200 in the right eye and counting fingers at five feet in the left eye. There was no improvement with pinhole in both eyes. He read four of eleven color plates with the right eye and only the test plate in the left eye. Pupils were sluggishly reactive bilaterally without an afferent pupillary defect. Anterior segment examination was remarkable for mild nuclear sclerotic cataract in both eyes, and posterior segment examination was remarkable for optic nerve pallor in both eyes.

Laboratory workup included vitamin A, folate, tsh, t4, folate, vit B1, CBC, basic metabolic profile, Lyme, RPR, and testing for Leber's hereditary optic neuropathy mutation. All were within normal limits.

MRI of the brain and orbits with and without contrast showed no mass. There were nonspecific white matter changes felt to be small vessel ischemic changes.

Humphrey visual field exam showed some superior altitudinal defects but interpretation was limited by the testing parameters.

OCT showed focal thinning in the papillomacular bundle in both eyes with normal retinal contour (Figs. 6.9 and 6.10).

He was advised to stop all alcohol and tobacco use. On a 2-month follow-up exam, his visual acuity with correction improved to 20/80 in the right eye and 20/400 in the left eye. On color vision testing, he was only able to read the test plate in each eye. His anterior and posterior segment exams were remarkable for mild nuclear sclerotic cataract and optic nerve pallor in both eyes.

OCT findings in tobacco alcohol amblyopia (TAA) have been previously published as case reports in the literature. Multiple reports describe an initial increase RNFL thickness

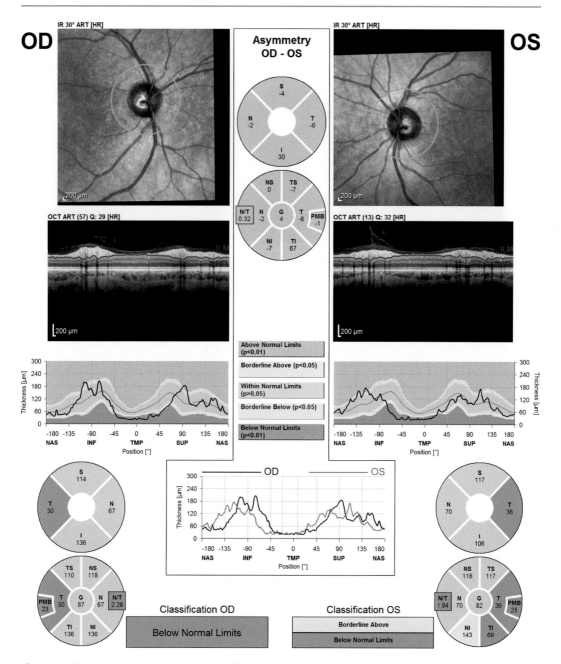

Fig. 6.9 OCT showed focal thinning in the papillomacular bundle in both eyes with normal retinal contour

with the exception of the temporal papillomacular bundle, which is within normal values or decreased. Over time, the RNFL thickness resolves at the areas of increased RNFL thickness and the temporal papillomacular bundle

shows thinning [17, 18]. These findings are similar to previously described findings in ethambutol toxicity. Although there are varying case reports on the OCT changes in ethambutol, one of the strongest studies followed

OD, IR 30° ART + OCT 30° (8.5 mm) ART (100) Q: 42 [HR]

OS, IR 30° ART + OCT 30° (8.6 mm) ART (100) Q: 42 [HR]

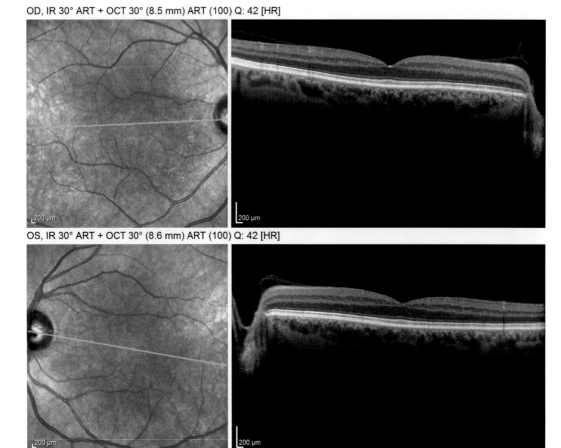

Fig. 6.10 OCT showed focal thinning in the papillomacular bundle in both eyes with normal retinal contour

52 patients (104 eyes) with OCT before, during, and after ethambutol therapy [19]. Only 3 of the 104 eyes showed OCT changes during treatment, but all of them had similar changes of temporal RNFL thinning [19]. In a smaller study of 20 eyes with optic neuropathy, no OCT changes were noted, but the study used time domain OCT [20]. The decreased resolution of time domain OCT may have been insufficient to identify the changes.

Case 5

A 55-year-old female with a history of hypertension, migraine, hyperlipidemia, hypothyroidism, and depression presented with vision in both eyes at near and far distances. She underwent cataract surgery 2 years prior in both eyes, which only mildly improved her vision.

Social history was positive for alcohol abuse and poor nutritional intake.

Her medications included gabapentin, sumatriptan, lisinopril, pravastatin, fluoxetine, quetiapine, and Synthroid.

Visual acuity was 20/50 in both eyes without any improvement on pinhole. She read 11 of 14 color plates in each eye and had briskly reactive pupils without an afferent pupillary defect.

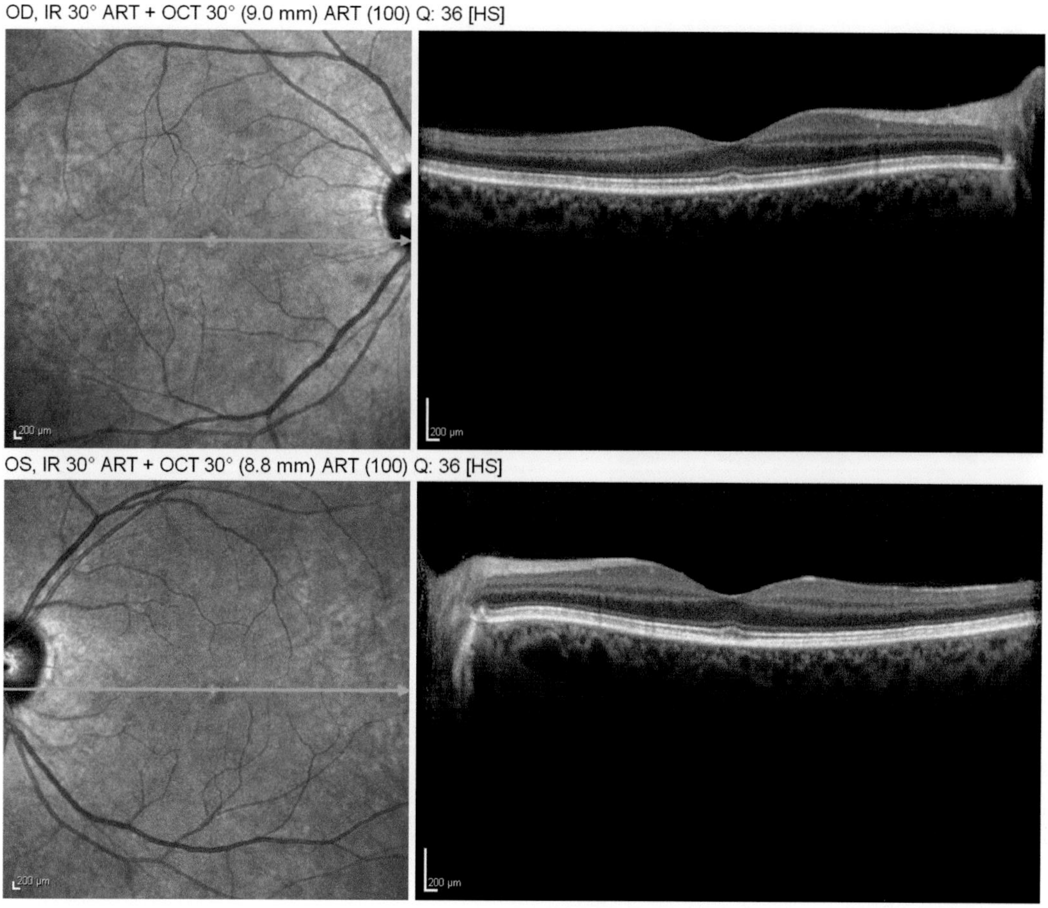

OD, IR 30° ART + OCT 30° (9.0 mm) ART (100) Q: 36 [HS]

OS, IR 30° ART + OCT 30° (8.8 mm) ART (100) Q: 36 [HS]

Fig. 6.11 There was additionally some discontinuity in the inner segment/outer segment line

Visual fields were full to confrontation and motility was full in both eyes. IOP was within normal limits and anterior exam was unremarkable except for well-positioned posterior chamber intraocular lenses. Posterior exam revealed a well-appearing optic nerve on the right and slight temporal thinning on the left, with mild changes in the retinal pigment epithelium in both eyes.

OCT showed bilateral symmetrical macular thinning extending from the peripheral posterior pole to the fovea with compression of the ellipsoid zone of the photoreceptors. There was additionally some discontinuity in the inner segment/outer segment line (Fig. 6.11). Her peripapillary retinal nerve fiber layer was normal (Fig. 6.12).

Laboratory workup revealed normal complete blood count, complete metabolic profile, folate, vitamin B12, vitamin A, RPR, Lyme antibodies, and MRI. Her vitamin B1 (thiamine) level was low and she was diagnosed with an optic neuropathy secondary to thiamine deficiency.

Wernicke encephalopathy, caused by thiamine deficiency, consists of the triad of ophthalmoplegia, confusion, and ataxia. While thiamine has also been associated with visual loss from optic neuropathy, there is a lack of reported OCT findings in the condition.

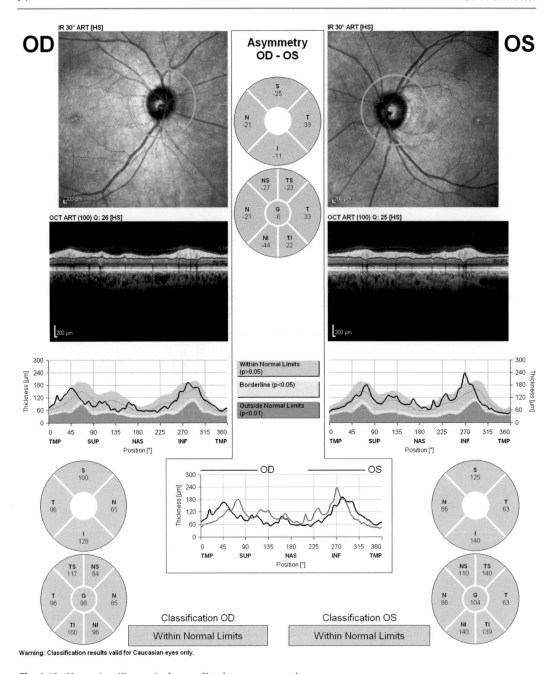

Fig. 6.12 Her peripapillary retinal nerve fiber layer was normal

References

1. Shinabarger D. Mechanism of action of the oxazolidinone antibacterial agents. Expert Opin Investig Drugs. 1999;8(8):1195–202. doi:10.1517/13543784.8.8.1195.
2. Kiuchi K, Miyashiro M, Kitagawa C, Wada S. Linezolid-associated optic neuropathy in a patient with ocular sarcoidosis. Jpn J Ophthalmol. 2009;53(4):420–4. doi:10.1007/s10384-009-0678-3.
3. Karuppannasamy D, Raghuram A, Sundar D. Linezolid-induced optic neuropathy. Indian J Ophthalmol. 2014;62(4):497–500. doi:10.4103/0301-4738.118451.
4. Joshi L, Taylor SRJ, Large O, Yacoub S, Lightman S. A case of optic neuropathy after short-term linezolid use in a patient with acute lymphocytic

leukemia. Clin Infect Dis. 2009;48(7):e73–4. doi:10.1086/597298.

5. Azamfirei L, Copotoiu S-M, Branzaniuc K, Szederjesi J, Copotoiu R, Berteanu C. Complete blindness after optic neuropathy induced by short-term linezolid treatment in a patient suffering from muscle dystrophy. Pharmacoepidemiol Drug Saf. 2007;16(4): 402–4. doi:10.1002/pds.1320.

6. Schecter GF, Scott C, True L, Raftery A, Flood J, Mase S. Linezolid in the treatment of multidrug-resistant tuberculosis. Clin Infect Dis. 2010;50(1): 49–55. doi:10.1086/648675.

7. Horwitz SB. Taxol (paclitaxel): mechanisms of action. Ann Oncol. 1994;5 Suppl 6:S3–6. Available at: http://www.ncbi.nlm.nih.gov/pubmed/7865431. Accessed 30 May 2014.

8. Capri G, Munzone E, Tarenzi E, et al. Optic nerve disturbances: a new form of paclitaxel neurotoxicity. J Natl Cancer Inst. 1994;86(14):1099–101. Available at: http://www.ncbi.nlm.nih.gov/pubmed/7912737.

9. Scaioli V, Caraceni A, Martini C, Curzi S, Capri G, Luca G. Electrophysiological evaluation of visual pathways in paclitaxel-treated patients. J Neurooncol. 2006;77(1):79–87. doi:10.1007/s11060-005-9008-x.

10. Lewis P, Waqar S, Yiannakis D, Raman V. Unilateral Optic Disc Papilloedema following Administration of Carboplatin Chemotherapy for Ovarian Carcinoma. Case Rep Oncol. 2014;7(1):29–32. doi:10.1159/000357912.

11. Bakbak B, Gedik S, Koktekir BE, et al. Assessment of ocular neurotoxicity in patients treated with systemic cancer chemotherapeutics. Cutan Ocul Toxicol. 2014;33(1):7–10. doi:10.3109/15569527.2013.787087.

12. Simon S, Athanasiov PA, Jain R, Raymond G, Gilhotra JS. Desferrioxamine-related ocular toxicity: a case report. Indian J Ophthalmol. 2012;60(4): 315–7. doi:10.4103/0301-4738.98714.

13. Baath JS, Lam W-C, Kirby M, Chun A. Deferoxamine-related ocular toxicity: incidence and outcome in a pediatric population. Retina. 2008;28(6):894–9. doi:10.1097/IAE.0b013e3181679f67.

14. Wong RW, Richa DC, Hahn P, Green WR, Dunaief JL. Iron toxicity as a potential factor in AMD. Retina. 2007;27(8):997–1003.

15. Ugarte M, Osborne NN, Brown LA, Bishop PN. Iron, zinc, and copper in retinal physiology and disease. Surv Ophthalmol. 2013;58(6):585–609. doi:10.1016/j.survophthal.2012.12.002.

16. Roth AM, Foos RY. Ocular pathologic changes in primary hemochromatosis. Arch Ophthalmol. 1972;87(5):507–14. Available at: http://www.ncbi.nlm.nih.gov/pubmed/5028091. Accessed 30 May 2014.

17. Bhatnagar A, Sullivan C. Tobacco-alcohol amblyopia: can OCT predict the visual prognosis? Eye (Lond). 2009;23(7):1616–8. doi:10.1038/eye.2008.285.

18. Kee C, Hwang J-M. Optical coherence tomography in a patient with tobacco-alcohol amblyopia. Eye (Lond). 2008;22(3):469–70. doi:10.1038/sj.eye.6702821.

19. Menon V, Jain D, Saxena R, Sood R. Prospective evaluation of visual function for early detection of ethambutol toxicity. Br J Ophthalmol. 2009;93(9):1251–4. doi:10.1136/bjo.2008.148502.

20. Kim U, Hwang J-M. Early stage ethambutol optic neuropathy: retinal nerve fiber layer and optical coherence tomography. Eur J Ophthalmol. 2009;19(3): 466–9. doi:. Available at: http://www.ncbi.nlm.nih.gov/pubmed/19396796. Accessed 30 May 2014.

Uveitis

7

Joan Lee

Abstract

There are many disorders inherent to the eye and others that are manifestation of systemic disease. The richly vascular uvea provides the connection from the body to the eye. Inflammation due to infection and autoimmune disease will manifest in the different parts of the uvea with secondary effects on other parts of the eye. Identification of the uveitides is challenging, and efforts are being made to standardize the categories of uveitis in efforts to create a systematic approach to this wide group of disorders. Because of the highly subjective nature of describing this group of diseases and the difficulty of optimal examinations in certain diseases, optical coherence tomography has provided an efficient, noninvasive way to identify and monitor one of the leading causes of vision loss in uveitis patients, macular disease.

Keywords

Macular edema • Epiretinal membrane • Chorioretinitis • Retinal vasculitis

The uvea comprises the middle coat of the eye and consists of the iris, ciliary body, and the choroid. Uveitis is a group of disorders that involves inflammation of the layers of the uvea. The etiology of inflammation ranges from infection and systemic immune disorders to iatrogenic causes. Identification and treatment of these disease processes can be complicated as the primary source of inflammation may not be clear. There has been extensive work among ophthalmologists to attempt to organize and classify the different types of uveitis. The International Uveitis Study Group (IUSG) and the Standardization of Uveitis Nomenclature (SUN) Working Group have made efforts to classify types of uveitis by anatomic location [1]. The SUN Working Group has established the main groups: anterior, intermediate, posterior, and panuveitis, determined clinically.

J. Lee, DO
Department of Ophthalmology, Geisinger Hospital, Danville, PA, USA
e-mail: joanjlee3@gmail.com

© Springer International Publishing Switzerland 2016
A. Girach, R.C. Sergott (eds.), *Optical Coherence Tomography*,
DOI 10.1007/978-3-319-24817-2_7

However, due to the level of clinical judgment in identifying disease processes, true standardization continues to be a challenge in this group of diseases with high visual morbidity.

Macular Edema

Macular edema is the leading cause of vision loss in uveitis patients [2]. It can be seen either directly as a result of macular infiltration or secondary to inflammation causing a disruption in the normal blood-retinal barrier and recruitment of inflammatory mediators: adenosine, prostaglandin E1, tumor necrosis factor alpha, interleukin 1 beta, vascular endothelial growth factor, and vasoactive peptides [2]. Prompt diagnosis is associated with more favorable visual outcomes. One study also reported a high rate of epiretinal membrane formation in patients with uveitic macular edema [3]. With the advent and development of optical coherence tomography (OCT), clinicians are able to follow primary or secondary posterior complications of uveitis objectively. OCT imaging also provides clinicians additional information which may be difficult to ascertain on clinical examination.

Anterior Uveitis

Anterior uveitis is the most common type of uveitis with the acute being the most common course. Causes include infectious, idiopathic, seronegative HLA-B27-associated arthropathies, juvenile idiopathic arthritis, and Fuch's heterochromic iridocyclitis, among many others [4]. Isolated anterior uveitis does not often have manifestations in the posterior segment of the eye. However, anterior uveitis may have posterior complications, most commonly macular edema (Fig. 7.1a). Anterior segment surgery (Fig. 7.1b) and medications have also been linked to cystoid macular edema, which is readily identified and can be monitored clinically or with OCT to look for response or progression.

Intermediate Uveitis

Intermediate uveitis is the least common form of uveitis. The most common causes include sarcoidosis, multiple sclerosis, Lyme disease, and idiopathic [4]. Vision loss from intermediate uveitis results from maculopathy, disc edema, and neovascularization. Clinically patients will demonstrate peripheral phlebitis, snow banking, neovascularization, disc edema, cystoid macular edema (Fig. 7.1c), and epiretinal membrane formation.

Posterior Uveitis

Posterior uveitis is the second most common form of uveitis. It is more commonly associated with infection than anterior or intermediate uveitis [4]. The most common cause of posterior uveitis is toxoplasmosis. Other common causes include cytomegalovirus, systemic lupus erythematosus, birdshot choroidopathy, and sarcoidosis, among others.

Toxoplasma gondii Obligate Intracellular Protozoan

Toxoplasma gondii, an obligate intracellular protozoan may be acquired congenitally or in the postnatal period. It often presents as a retinochoroiditis. In newborns, associated systemic disease may be identified, including anemia, rash, thrombocytopenia, hepatitis, hepatosplenomegaly, pneumonitis, encephalitis, and myocarditis [4]. Most patients who acquire this systemic infection in the postnatal period are asymptomatic or have a mild course. If patients are visually symptomatic, the symptoms reported are most commonly blurred vision and floaters [4]. Retinochoroiditis is often recurrent and develop at the margins of old scars [4]. Acute lesions are typically yellow gray in color clinically and involve the superficial retina with surrounding edema (Fig. 7.2a). Vitritis and retinal vascular occlusions may be present as well as perivascu-

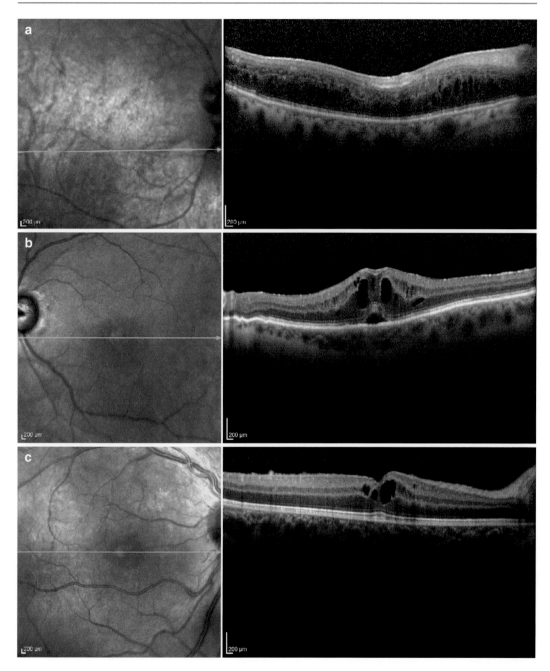

Fig. 7.1 Different patterns of macular edema in uveitis. (**a**) Diffuse macular edema in psoriatic arthritis with multifocal choroiditis. (**b**) Pseudophakic cystoid macular edema with serous detachment (**c**). Cystoid macular edema in pars planitis

lar exudates and arteriolar plaques [4, 5]. Over time the lesion becomes more distinct and creates a pigmented chorioretinal scar (Fig. 7.2b, c). The chorioretinal scars, which are often seen in congenital disease, have well-defined borders with central atrophy and peripheral RPE hyperplasia [4]. OCT is being utilized to understand the morphologic features of the disease. A pro-

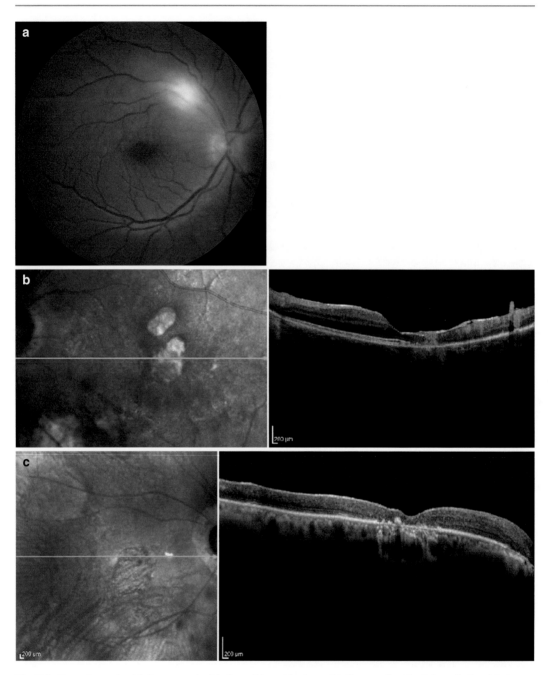

Fig. 7.2 Toxoplasmosis. (**a**) Acute acquired lesion with associated chorioretinal thickening. (**b**) Focal area of macular thinning and scar formation. (**c**) Diffuse macular thinning with increased reflectivity of choroid due to retinal atrophy in a patient from Brazil

spective observational study of 15 patients with active ocular toxoplasmosis identified increased retinal reflectivity and RPE choriocapillaris/choroidal optical shadowing at the active site. Twenty-four weeks later there was evidence of resolution of the disease demonstrated on OCT as disorganized retinal signal and thickness. Authors suggest that OCT may be helpful in identifying disease activity which may aid in treatment algorithms [6].

Systemic Infections

Systemic infections manifest in the eye due to the rich circulation of the uvea. Infectious chorioretinitis or endophthalmitis may result from a variety of infectious organisms. Candida endophthalmitis can cause an initial retinochoroiditis that may develop into an endophthalmitis by breaking through the retina into the vitreous [4]. Risk factors for candida endophthalmitis include recent hospitalization, diabetes mellitus, liver disease, renal failure, cancer, indwelling catheters, systemic surgery, organ transplantation, HIV/AIDS, IV drug use, hyperalimentation, and immunosuppressive drugs [7, 8]. Patients may be asymptomatic and complain of pain, redness, floaters, and vision loss [4]. Often located in the posterior pole, the lesions can be multiple and are white and deep on clinical examination (Fig. 7.3). They may have associated white-centered hemorrhages and nerve fiber layer infarcts [4]. These lesions can be followed as they progress to chorioretinal scars and may help in determining response to antifungal treatment.

Syphilis

Syphilis is caused by a spirochetal bacterial infection by *Treponema pallidum*. It is a sexually transmitted disease, which boasts the title "great imitator" due to its ability to mimic other systemic and ocular disease. Syphilis can present in four stages, primary, secondary, latent, and tertiary. The primary stage manifests with a chancre. The secondary phase presents with rash and lymphadenopathy. The latent phase presents with no systemic disease, and the tertiary stage presents with cardiovascular problems, neurosyphilis, and gummas (granulomatous

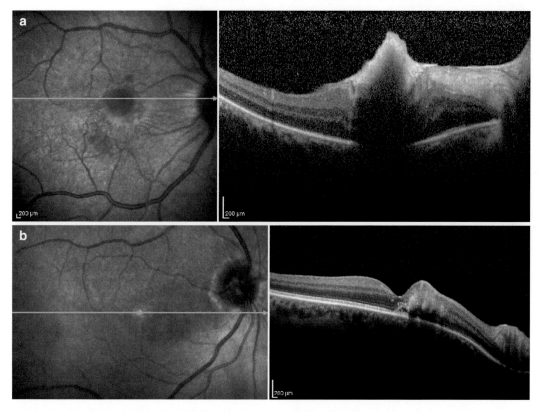

Fig. 7.3 Fungal endophthalmitis. (**a**) Hyper-reflective outer retina with shadowing of underlying choroid and retina which had seeded into the vitreous in a 34-year-old patient with history of intravenous drug use. (**b**) Chorioretinal lesion seen in a 55-year-old with history of alcohol abuse

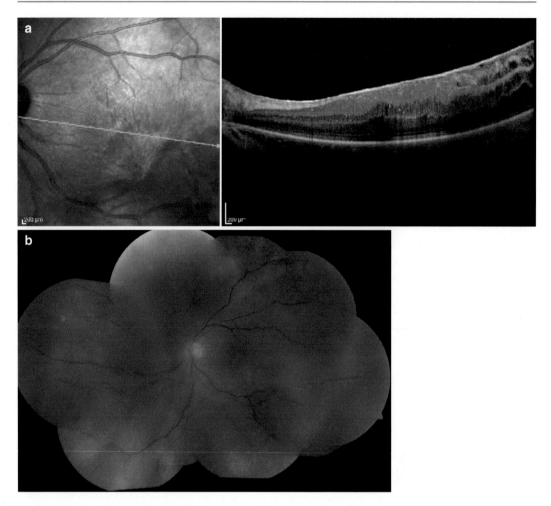

Fig. 7.4 Syphilis. (**a**) Epiretinal membrane formation 3 months after treatment for panuveitis. (**b**) Preretinal fibrosis and tractional detachment inferotemporal

lesions which can be located anywhere on the body). It can affect all parts of the eye and uveitis is the most common presentation of ocular disease [4]. Patients may have varied presentations including chorioretinitis, panuveitis, vitritis, keratic precipitates, vascular sheathing, optic disc edema, intermediate uveitis, exudative retinal detachments, and necrotizing retinitis [4, 9]. Chorioretinitis is the most common form of syphilitic posterior involvement [4]. Ophthalmic involvement is a sign of tertiary syphilis particularly when the optic nerve and retina are involved [9]. The route of treatment for ocular involvement includes both intramuscular injections of penicillin for 3 weeks and IV penicillin for 10–14 days. Ocular complications include cataracts,

glaucoma, macular edema, epiretinal membranes, proliferative vitreoretinopathy, and retinal traction [4] (Fig. 7.4a, b).

White Dot Syndromes

The white dot syndromes are a group of inflammatory disorders that affect the posterior segment of the eye. Included in this group are acute posterior multifocal placoid pigment epitheliopathy (APMPPE), birdshot chorioretinopathy, diffuse unilateral subacute neuroretinitis (DUSN), multiple evanescent white dot syndrome (MEWDS), multifocal choroiditis with panuveitis (MFS), serpiginous choroiditis, punctate inner choroiditis

(PIC), subretinal fibrosis and uveitis syndrome, acute zonal occult outer retinopathy (AZOOR), and acute retinal pigment epitheliitis [10, 11].

Acute Posterior Multifocal Placoid Pigment Epitheliopathy

Acute posterior multifocal placoid pigment epitheliopathy is a bilateral white dot syndrome that often affects healthy young individuals. Symptoms include blurred vision, scotomas, and photopsias. Viral association and etiology have been hypothesized. Yellowish placoid lesions are at the level of the retinal pigment epithelium (Fig. 7.5).

Choroidal nonperfusion is suggested as the primary cause [10, 11]. There have been rare cases associated with CNS vasculitis [12]. OCT highlights the location of pathology in this disorder and may help identify this disorder in atypical cases.

Birdshot Chorioretinopathy

Birdshot chorioretinopathy described by both Gass and Maumenee is a bilateral white dot syndrome with strong association with HLA-A29 [13]. Symptoms include blurred vision, floaters, photopsias, and impaired night vision and color

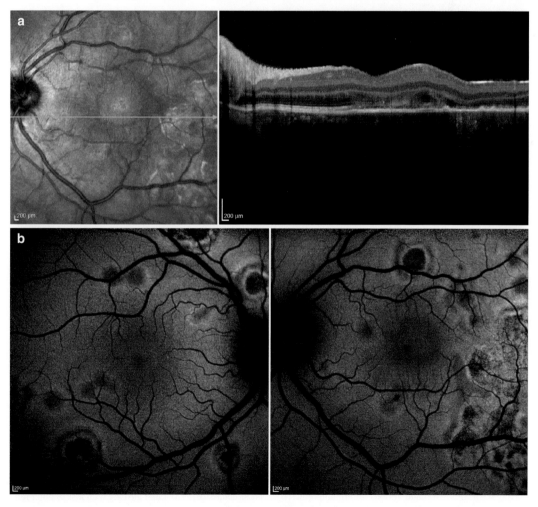

Fig. 7.5 Acute posterior multifocal placoid pigment epitheliopathy (APMPPE). (**a**) Disease activity seen at the level of RPE. (**b**) Hypofluorescent areas of retinal pigment epithelial atrophy with surrounding rings of hyperfluorescence indicating excess lipofuscin from dysfunctional RPE cells

vision [11]. Yellow-orange lesions radiate from the optic nerve and are associated with vitritis (Fig. 7.6a). Retinal vasculitis (Fig. 7.6b), macular edema, epiretinal membrane, disc edema, and choroidal neovascularization are some complications [4, 10, 11]. Optic, macular, and chorioretinal atrophy have been implicated as the cause of visual morbidity in this disorder. Recent studies have illustrated that the outer retinal thinning is the major cause of macular thinning in birdshot chorioretinopathy [14] (Fig. 7.6c, d).

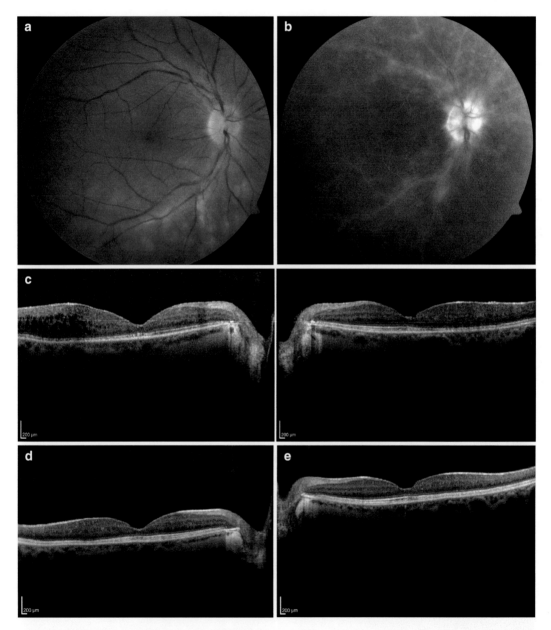

Fig. 7.6 Birdshot chorioretinopathy. (**a**) Fundus photo of classic deep yellow-orange lesions inferotemporal. (**b**) Fluorescein angiography with retinal vasculitis. (**c**) OCT in the same patient with epiretinal membrane formation on right causing temporal macular edema, loss of retinal architecture. (**d**, **e**) Macular atrophy with loss of outer retinal anatomy

Serpiginous Choroiditis

Serpiginous choroiditis is a bilateral asymmetric, chronic, and progressive white dot syndrome which typically affects older individuals in their sixth and seventh decade of life [4]. Symptoms include blurred vision, metamorphopsia, and scotomata. A yellow-gray deep lesion is seen on fundoscopy extending in a pseudopodial pattern often in a peripapillary location [4] (Fig. 7.7a). Inflammation is seen at the edge of the lesion. The disease is resistant to treatment. Findings on OCT illustrate destruction of the retinal pigment epithelial layer [2] (Fig. 7.7b).

Sarcoidosis

Sarcoidosis is a granulomatous disorder that primarily involves the lungs, skin, eyes, and lymph nodes. Diagnosis is based on demonstrating non-caseating granulomas in a tissue biopsy. Ocular involvement can occur at virtually any age and can affect any part of the eye. It is more severe in the African American population. Steroids are the mainstay of treatment [4]. Macular involvement is, again, a large cause of vision loss, from cystoid macular degeneration to epiretinal membrane formation (Fig. 7.8).

Retinal Vasculitides

Retinal vasculitides are another group of inflammatory disorders that affect the retinal blood vessels. They may involve the arteries or veins and cause a sheathing of the blood vessels when examined clinically. Often there is accompanying inflammation in other parts of the eye. It may be a manifestation of systemic disease. Behcet's disease was found to be the most common cause of retinal vasculitis in a recent study [15]. Other causes include Eales' disease, idiopathic retinal vasculitis, aneurysms and neuroretinitis syndrome (IRVAN), frosted branch angiitis, multiple sclerosis, Susac's syndrome, sarcoidosis, Buerger's disease, inflammatory bowel disease, rheumatoid disease, HLA-B27-associated uveitis, Sjogren's syndrome, systemic lupus erythematosus, ANCA-associated vasculitides, polyarteritis nodosa, tuberculosis, syphilis, cat scratch disease, toxoplasmosis, Epstein-Barr virus, cytomegalovirus, herpes simplex and zoster virus, human immunodeficiency virus, drug-induced retinal vasculitis, cancer-associated retinopathy, and intraocular lymphoma [4]. Symptoms include painless loss of vision, scotomas, and floaters. Both eyes are affected in all cases [4]. The complications of retinal vasculitis include neovascularization, retinal and macular ischemia, and non-ophthalmic manifestations of occlusive disease if part of a systemic disorder.

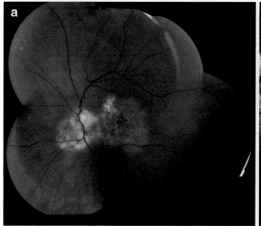
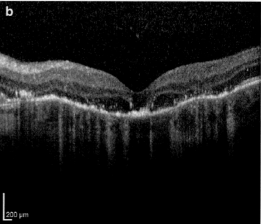

Fig. 7.7 Serpiginous choroiditis. (**a**) Fundus photo with deep yellow-gray lesion located in the classic peripapillary location with pseudopodial pattern. (**b**) Destruction of the RPE layer with atrophy

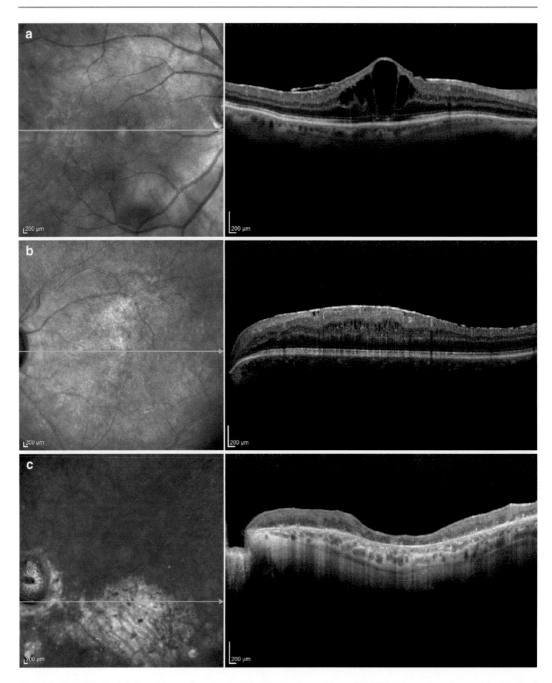

Fig. 7.8 Sarcoidosis. (**a**) Cystoid macular edema with epiretinal membrane. (**b**) Diffuse macular edema with epiretinal membrane. (**c**) Diffuse macular atrophy

Susac's Syndrome

Susac's syndrome, first described in 1979, is a rare occlusive arterial disease that affects the brain, eye, and ear. Patients typically present with vision loss from multiple branch retinal artery occlusions (Fig. 7.9a, b), progressive hearing loss and a variety of neurologic symptoms. The neurologic symptoms may range from depression, memory loss, to hemiparesis and often are the most severe symptoms of the disease. MRI is the imaging modality of choice and will show lesions of the corpus callosum [16] (Fig. 7.9c). The disease course is chronic and relapsing, and all symptoms may not present at the same time which makes diagnosis difficult. OCT and retinal imaging modalities can help establish the diagnosis of retinal vascular occlusive disease which could be missed on initial ophthalmoscopic examination.

Masquerade Syndromes

The masquerade syndromes should also be considered in the investigation of posterior uveitis. Cancer-associated retinopathy and ocular lymphoma can have posterior segment findings and retinal vascular changes which may be difficult to follow clinically. CNS lymphoma may initially be unilateral but is almost always a bilateral disease. There may be mild

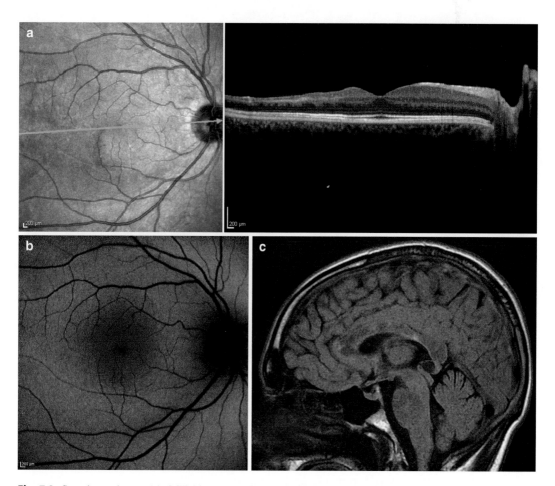

Fig. 7.9 Susac's syndrome. (**a**) OCT illustrates diffuse full-thickness retinal atrophy at the level of the branch retinal artery occlusion. (**b**) Fundus autofluorescence highlights the abrupt loss of retinal arterial vasculature along the inferior arcade (**c**). MRI T2 Flair sagittal image illustrates hyperintense lesions in the corpus callosum

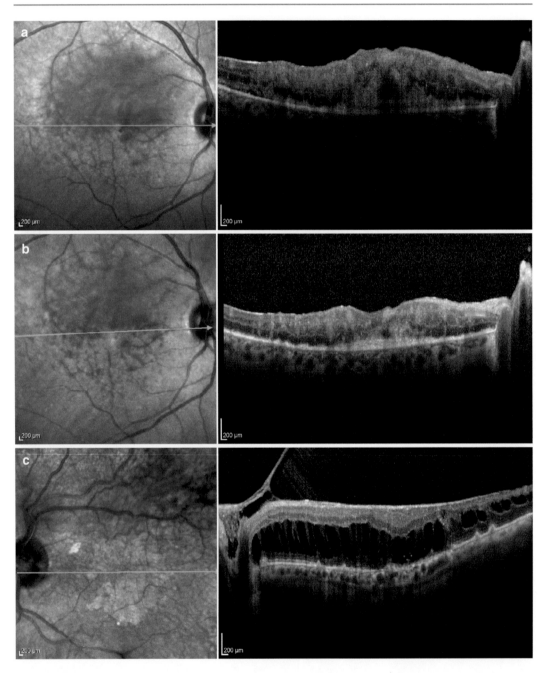

Fig. 7.10 CNS lymphoma. (**a**) Retinal infiltrative lesion with hyperdense subretinal lesion in a 58-year-old woman with known history of diffuse large B cell lymphoma. (**b**) Five days following intravitreal methotrexate, improved retinal thickening, and subretinal lesion. (**c**) Tractional retinal detachment in a different patient with CNS lymphoma

inflammation seen on clinical exam with large multifocal yellow lesions with pigment epithelial detachment [4]. Although diagnosis requires histopathologic identification of malignant cells, OCT can be used to quantitatively follow the progression of disease or response to treatment (Fig. 7.10a, b) and complications (Fig. 7.10c).

Conclusions

As a vascular structure, the uvea serves as an important source of nutrition for the eye while also serving as a protective barrier. Because it serves as a connection to the rest of the body through systemic blood supply, there are infinite conditions that can be manifest in the eye through the uvea and secondarily in the retina. Inflammation breaks down the blood-retinal barrier and may also allow infections to penetrate the retina and vitreous through the middle coat of the eye. Often these patients have symptoms of pain and stigmata of inflammation in the anterior parts of the eye which makes consistent posterior examinations limited and subjective. Macular disease is one of the most common causes of vision loss in patients with uveitis. Due to the level of visual morbidity of this large group of ophthalmic disease, OCT has proven to be an indispensable tool to provide objective data to identify and monitor disease.

References

1. Jabs DA, Nussenblatt RB, Rosenbaum JT, Standardization of Uveitis Nomenclature (SUN) Working Group. Standardization of uveitis nomenclature for reporting clinical data. Results of the First International Workshop. Am J Ophthalmol. 2005;140:509–16.
2. Gallagher MJ, Yilmaz T, Cervantes-Castaneda RA. The characteristic features of optical coherence tomography in posterior uveitis. Br J Ophthalmol. 2007;91:1680–5.
3. Markomichelakis NN, Halkiadakis I, Pantelia E, Peponis V, Patelis A, Theodossiadis P, Theodossiadis G. Patterns of macular edema in patients with uveitis: qualitative and quantitative assessment using optical coherence tomography. Ophthalmology. 2004;111:946–53.
4. Foster SC, Vitale AT. Diagnosis and treatment of uveitis. 2nd ed. New Delhi: Jaypee Brothers Medical Publishing; 2013.
5. Holland GN. Ocular toxoplasmosis: a global reassessment. Part II: disease manifestations and management. Am J Ophthlamol. 2004;137:1–17.
6. Orefice JL, Costa RA, Orefice F. Vitreoretinal morphology in active ocular toxoplasmosis: a prospective study by optical coherence tomography. Br J Ophthalmol. 2007;91:773–80.
7. Shrader SK, Band JD, Lauter CB, Murphy P. The clinical spectrum of endophthalmitis: incidence predisposing factors, and features influencing outcome. J Infect Dis. 1990;162(1):115–20.
8. Essman TF, Flynn Jr HW, Smiddy WE, Brod RD, Murray TG, Davis JL, Rubsamen PE. Treatment outcomes in a 10 year study of endogenous fungal endophthalmitis. Ophthalmic Surg Lasers. 1997;28:185–94.
9. Chao JR, Khurana RN, Fawzi AA, Reddy HS, Rao NA. Syphilis: reemergence of an old adversary. Ophthalmology. 2006;113:2074–9.
10. Quillen DA, Davis JB, Gottlieb JL, Blodi BA, Callanan DG, Chang TS, Equi RA. The white dot syndromes. Am J Ophthalmol. 2004;137:538–50.
11. Moorthy RS, Roa PK, Read RW, et al. Basic and Clinical Science Course (BCSC): intraocular inflammation and uveitis. San Francisco: American Academy of Ophthalmology; 2011.
12. Wilson CA, Choromokos EA, Sheppard R. Acute posterior multifocal placoid pigment epitheliopathy and cerebral vasculitis. Arch Ophthalmol. 1988;106:796–800.
13. Nussenblatt RB, Mittal KK, Ryan S, Green WR, Maumenee AE. Birdshot retinochoroidopathy associated with HLA-A29 antigen and immune responsiveness to retinal S-antigen. Am J Ophthalmol. 1982;113:33–5.
14. Birch DG, Williams PD, Callanan D, Wang R, Locke KG, Hood DC. Macular atrophy in birdshot retinochoroidopathy: an optical coherence tomography and multifocal electroretinography analysis. Retina. 2010;30:930–7.
15. Mili-Boussen I, Letaief I, Zbiba W, Trabelsi O, Ben Younes N, Abid J, et al. Retinal vasculitis. Epidemiological, clinical and etiological features. J Fr Opthalmol. 2010;59:297–301.
16. O'Halloran HS, Pearson PA, Lee WB, Susac JO, Berger JR. Microangiopathy of the brain, retina and cochlea (Susac syndrome). Ophthalmology. 1988;105:1038–44.

Glaucoma and Other Optic Neuropathies

8

Teri T. Kleinberg

Abstract

Optic neuropathies are characterized by specific patterns of damage to the ganglion cells and retinal nerve fiber layer. The reproducibility of spectral-domain optical coherence tomography (SD-OCT) has allowed for objective measurement and tracking of these patterns of damage. This chapter reviews major types of optic neuropathies including glaucoma, optic neuritis, disc edema, anterior ischemic optic neuropathy, disc drusen, diabetic papillitis, and Lyme papillitis.

Keywords

Glaucoma • Optic neuritis • Disc drusen • Papilledema • Ischemic optic neuropathy • Giant cell arteritis

Optic neuropathies result in damage to the retinal nerve fiber layer and are characterized by differing time courses and patterns of damage. We are fortunate that the reproducibility of SD-OCT has permitted the quantification of pattern and degree of damage in order to distinguish between pathologies. For example, anterior ischemic optic neuropathy, optic disc drusen, and glaucoma all share a predilection for superior and inferior retinal nerve fiber layer (RNFL) loss, while other nonglaucomatous optic neuropathies cause loss of the temporal RNFL [1]. OCT has become a key adjunct to the clinical exam. Discussed in this chapter, with case studies to illustrate, are multiple optic neuropathies including glaucoma, optic neuritis, disc edema, anterior ischemic optic neuropathy, disc drusen, diabetic papillitis, and Lyme papillitis.

Glaucoma

Glaucoma is a progressive optic neuropathy resulting in loss of the retinal ganglion cells and their axons [2]. The pathogenesis of glaucoma is damage to the retinal ganglion cells that results anatomically in retinal nerve fiber layer thinning and functionally in lost photoreceptor sensitivity manifested through changes in visual field testing.

T.T. Kleinberg, MD, MSc
Department of Neuro-Ophthalmology,
Wills Eye Hospital, Philadelphia, PA, USA
e-mail: terikleinberg@gmail.com

Pre-perimetric Glaucoma

There is great value in diagnosing glaucoma prior to changes on visual field testing. Often, patients present with suspicious clinical findings such as optic disc cupping, and it is a great challenge to decide on the diagnosis of glaucoma or the timing of treatment initiation. By 1991, it was already known from careful evaluation of optic disc photographs that a majority of eyes had RNFL loss at least 5 years preceding visual field changes [3]. OCT has recently been shown to demonstrate RNFL loss prior to detectable visual field changes [4].

Macular Changes

The highest density of retinal ganglion cells is in the macula, where ganglion cells and RNFL make up approximately 1/3 of the total retinal thickness. In glaucoma monitoring, the parameter that is routinely measured is RNFL loss, which is a proxy for damage to retinal ganglion cells. Direct measurement of reduction in macular thickness could be an additional diagnostic parameter for identifying early glaucoma on OCT [5, 6]. Significant changes between the normal macula and the early glaucomatous macula, particularly in the outer temporal macula, have been demonstrated [5]. Even early in the disease process, macular damage is present [7]. There is a robust structure-function relationship between the rate of macular thinning and progression of visual loss [8–10]. With the high-resolution imaging obtainable from modern OCT, early patterns of retinal ganglion cell loss can be detected and monitored for change over time. Hood and colleagues showed that there is greater glaucomatous thinning in the inferior retina corresponding to the superior visual field [7]. Macular damage from glaucoma is typically arcuate in nature and associated with local RNFL thinning, with particularly dramatic thinning of the inferior region of the macula projecting to a small area of the inferotemporal

disc referred to as the "macular vulnerability zone" [7].

Cases

Figure 8.1 is from a 90-year-old African American male who was lost to follow-up for several years with advanced glaucoma. His vision was 20/25 OD and no light perception OS. He was pseudophakic after a cataract extraction and trabeculectomy OD for pressures not controlled with drops. Field testing revealed only a small central island of vision remaining OD. OCT shows severe RNFL loss bilaterally, with the only remaining areas of thickness approaching normal at vascular bundles.

Figure 8.2 shows a 65-year-old Caucasian male who presented with bilateral blurry vision and was found to have advanced open angle glaucoma. He had a strong family history of glaucoma. Humphrey visual fields demonstrated superior arcuate changes OD and general depression OS. Goldmann visual fields were performed, and he was found to have full field OD and inferior deficit OS. OCT showed enlarged cup to disc bilaterally with deep cups. Macular thickness was also decreased, with flattened foveal and macular contours consistent with a bilateral optic neuropathy.

Figure 8.3 shows an 80-year-old African American female with normal tension open angle glaucoma. Her vision is 20/25 OU with mild nuclear sclerotic cataracts. Her optic discs show cupping OU with superior and inferior narrowing OD and inferior narrowing OS (Fig. 8.3a). Humphrey visual fields show a stable superior nasal step and inferior arcuate defect OD and a superior arcuade defect OS with paracentral visual field loss (Fig. 8.3b). OCT shows superior, nasal, and inferior RNFL thinning OD and inferotemporal thinning OS (Fig. 8.3c). Although there is asymmetric RNFL loss, with the appearance of more significant loss OD, the small inferotemporal band of RNFL loss OS affects the central vision and causes more visual disability. This is also shown in the macular thickness maps from the same time point (Fig. 8.3d).

Fig. 8.1 Advanced open angle glaucoma. FoDi shows severe RNFL loss bilaterally with artificial normal measurements at vascular bundles only

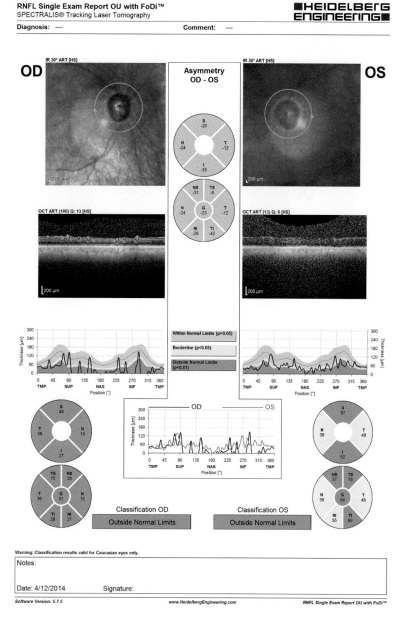

Optic Neuritis

Typical Optic Neuritis: Multiple Sclerosis

As the RNFL is composed nearly entirely of axons, the retina provides an opportunity to assess axonal loss in multiple sclerosis (MS) using OCT to provide quantitative measurements.

Retinal axonal loss presents early in the course of multiple sclerosis and becomes increasingly prominent in more advanced stages of the disease. Even eyes of MS patients without a previous optic neuritis have reduction in RNFL and macular volume as compared to healthy controls [11]. RNFL thinning and reduction of macular volume are most prominent in eyes previously affected by optic neuritis and are associated with greater disease severity and greater cortical gray matter atrophy [12]. Patients with a clinically isolated syndrome (CIS), the first clinical demyelinating attack suggestive of multiple sclerosis, have been shown to have total and temporal peripapillary RNFL thinning but no difference in macular volume as compared to controls [13]. In

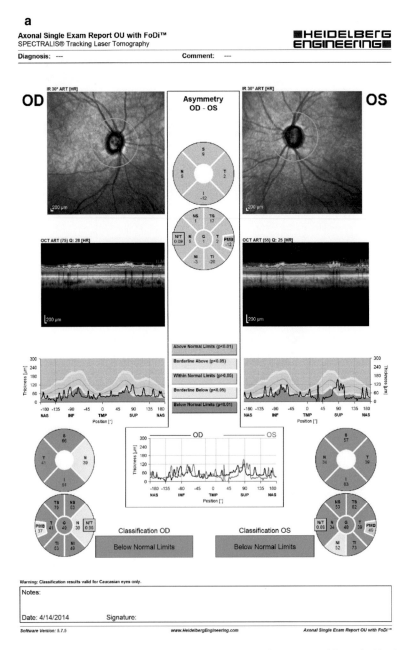

Fig. 8.2 Advanced open angle glaucoma. (**a**) FoDi RNFL map showed decreased peripapillary RNFL thickness in all quadrants of both eyes. (**b**) Macular thickness heat-maps demonstrate bilateral thinning with more macular thinning in the superior macula OS on the asymmetry analysis as compared to OD

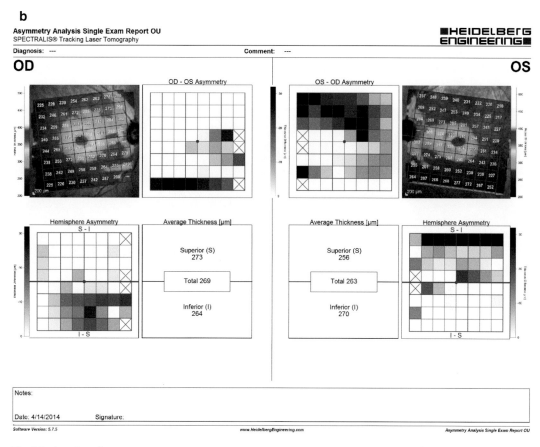

Fig. 8.2 (continued)

advanced disease, both with and without a history of optic neuritis, there is a pattern of temporal-predominant peripapillary RNFL thinning, which contains fibers of the papillomacular bundle [13]. As the severity of MS progresses, RFNL thinning becomes increasingly prominent: secondary progressive MS>relapsing-remitting MS>CIS [11, 13]. This is most pronounced in eyes affected by symptomatic optic neuritis. Therefore, OCT has the potential to be used as a quantitative marker of axonal injury for use both in patient care and treatment research.

Figure 8.4 shows a 36-year-old male with a prior history of multiple sclerosis who was seen in follow-up 4 weeks after an optic neuritis flare in the right eye when he presented with 20/400 vision OD. His vision is 20/25 OD and 20/20 OS. He had bilateral progressive RNFL thinning

and flattening of the foveal and macular contours over the previous 3 years.

Atypical Optic Neuritis

Neuromyelitis optica (NMO), also known as Devic's disease, is an inflammatory, demyelinating condition of the central nervous system causing optic neuritis and transverse myelitis associated with antibodies against aquaporin-4 molecules (aquaporin-4 immunoglobulin G, NMO-IgG). Patients have multiple episodes of optic neuritis with resultant RNFL thinning.

Differences in RNFL thickness may help differentiate between types of optic neuritis, including relapsing-remitting multiple sclerosis (RRMS), chronic relapsing inflammatory optic neuritis (CRION), and neuromyelitis optica (NMO). According to a recent study, an RNFL of 41 μm is 100 % specific for optic neuritis associated with NMO and CRION as compared to RRMS [14]. RRMS has substantially thicker RNFL than patients with NMO or CRION.

Figure 8.5 is from a 36-year-old African American female presented with gradual decrease in vision in the left eye to count fingers vision over 6 months. She had been recently

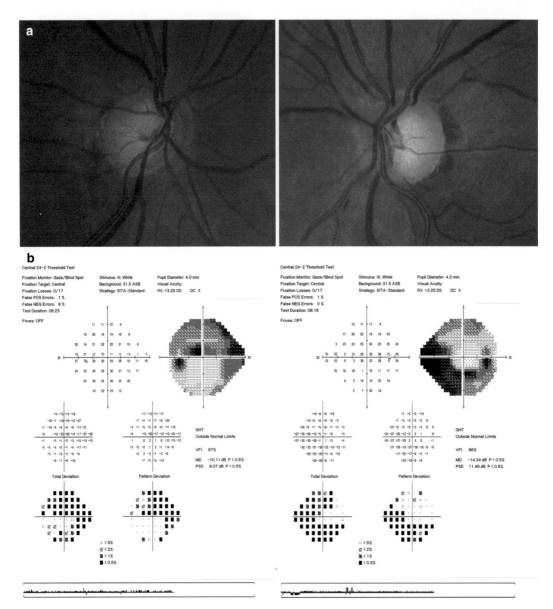

Fig. 8.3 Normal tension open angle glaucoma. (**a**) Optic disc photos. (**b**) Humphrey visual fields. OD shows superior nasal step and inferior arcuate defect. OS shows superior and paracentral visual field loss. (**c**) FoDi RNFL map at time point corresponding to visual fields shown in (**b**). There is asymmetric thinning of the RNFL, with superior, nasal, and temporal thinning OD and inferotemporal thinning OS. (**d**) Macular thickness map comparison at the same time point as (**c**). Greater RNFL loss in the inferotemporal sector OS causes marked asymmetry in the overall macular thickness heat maps and has a greater effect on central vision. The OS map clearly demonstrates the widespread inferior macular thinning seen with damage to the macular vulnerability zone at the inferotemporal optic nerve

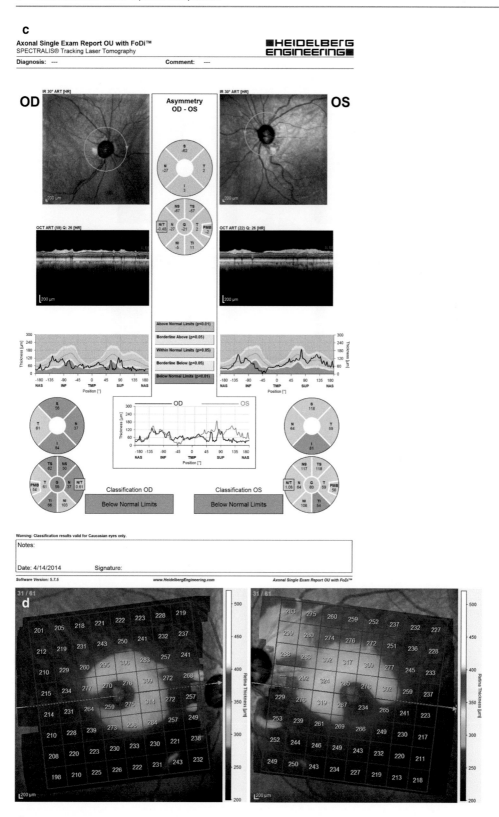

Fig. 8.3 (continued)

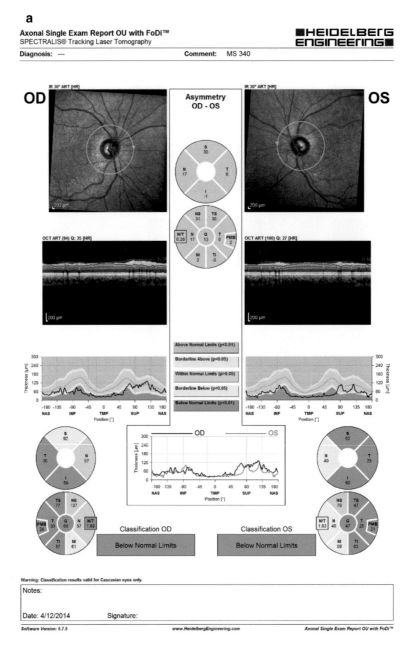

Fig. 8.4 Multiple sclerosis. (**a**) FoDi RNFL map showing bilateral thinning on presentation at age 31. (**b**) FoDi RNFL maps showing progressive bilateral thinning on a follow-up at age 36. (**c**) Right eye posterior pole macular thickness change and hemisphere asymmetry maps demonstrating change over a 1-year period. There is significant hemispheric asymmetry, with more loss throughout the inferior macula than superiorly

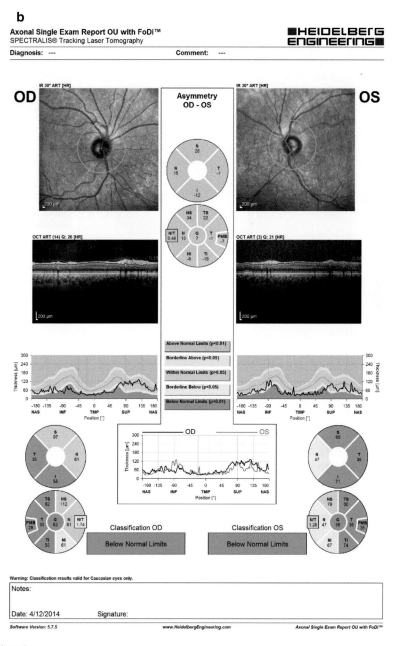

Fig. 8.4 (continued)

c

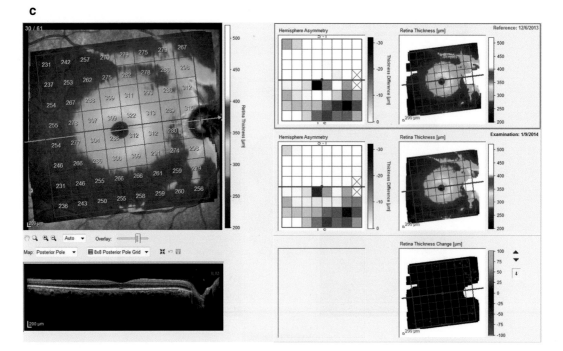

Fig. 8.4 (continued)

diagnosed with sarcoidosis with lung involvement. She had a dense left relative afferent papillary defect. Fundus exam revealed disc edema and a large macular choroidal granuloma with serous retinal detachment. Contrast-enhanced MRI of the brain and orbits showed enhancement of the posterior aspect of the left globe and anterior optic nerve. Initial OCT (Fig. 8.5a) demonstrates normal peripapillary retinal nerve fiber layer thickness in the right eye. In the left eye, there is significant retinal nerve fiber layer thickening and some areas of detachment of the optic disc to the peripapillary retina, demonstrating optic disc edema. Three-month follow-up demonstrates persistent but reduced RNFL thickening consistent with disc edema (Fig. 8.5b). Resolution of macular subretinal fluid over the three-month period could also clearly be seen on macular line scans (Fig. 8.5c–e).

Disc Edema

OCT can be used to aid in distinguishing between true disc edema and pseudopapilledema including disc drusen and can be used to follow resolution of disc edema over time. Classically, the clinical findings of disc edema are optic disc hyperemia, peripapillary retinal nerve fiber hemorrhages, peripapillary retinal nerve fiber layer edema, distention of retinal veins, loss of spontaneous pulsations of the retinal veins near the optic disc, and disc elevation [15]. On OCT, the peripapillary RNFL is thickened beyond the upper limit of normal. Subretinal and intraretinal fluid can also be seen tracking into the macula. There is a hyporeflective space between the sensory retina and the retinal pigment epithelium and choriocapillaris complex that has been called the subretinal hyporeflective space (SHYPS) [16]. The SHYPS has been noted to form a "lazy V" pattern in disc edema (Fig. 8.7).

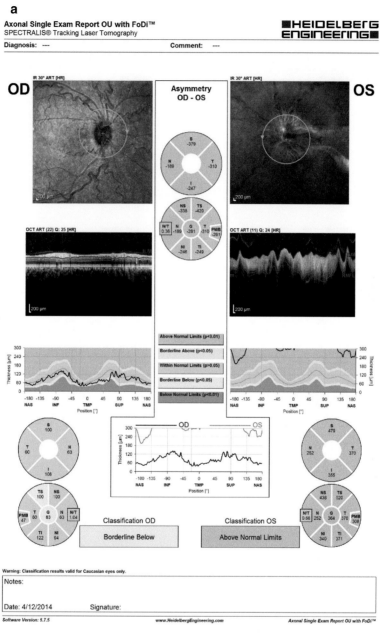

Fig. 8.5 Atypical optic neuritis. (**a**) Initial presentation of sarcoid optic neuritis with dramatic RNFL thickening. (**b**) Follow-up of sarcoid optic neuritis after 3 months. Note interval reduction in RNFL edema in the left eye, while right eye appears stable. (**c**) Macular line scan of left eye showing infrared image to the left and line scan to the right. There is dramatic detachment of the peripapillary retina into the fovea in addition to microcystic edema in the inner nuclear layer. (**d**) Normal right eye infrared image (*left*) and macular line scan (*right*) on patient presentation for comparison. (**e**) Interval resolution of sub-retinal fluid in the left eye at 3-month follow-up with consolidation and contraction of the retina

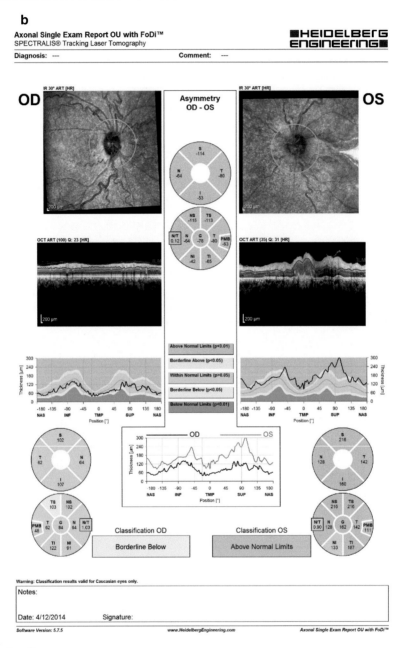

Fig. 8.5 (continued)

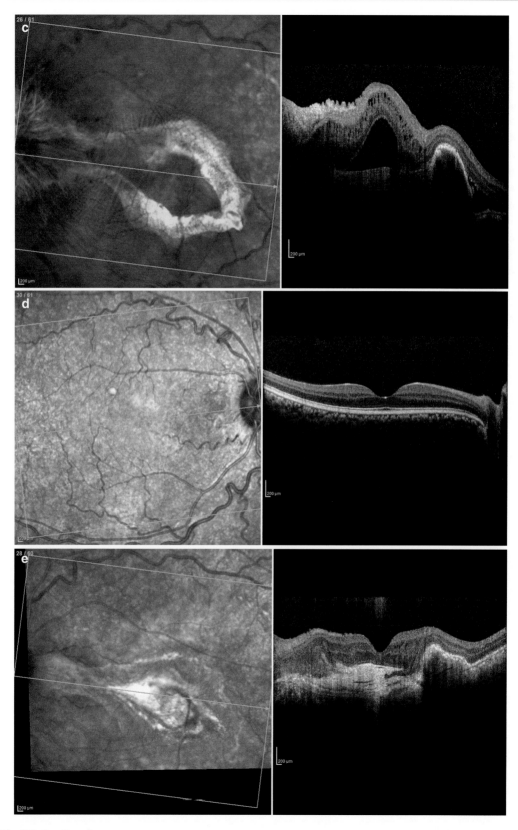

Fig. 8.5 (continued)

Figure 8.6 shows a 23-year-old African American female presented with 2 weeks of blurry vision OU, headache, pulsatile tinnitus, and occasional transient visual obscurations. Her vision was 20/100 OU. She was found to have bilateral disc edema. A lumbar puncture showed elevated opening pressure of 38 cm of water. MRI and magnetic resonance venography (MRV) were normal. She was started on oral prednisone and acetazolamide. Pupils were brisk with no relative afferent papillary defect. Color plates were reduced at 8/11 OD and 5/11 OS. Humphrey visual fields (HVF) showed characteristic enlargement of the blind spot in both eyes (Fig. 8.6a). Initial OCT (Fig. 8.6b) showed bilateral optic disc edema as well as subfoveal

edema in both eyes. Her vision and symptoms improved over 2 weeks corresponding to improvements in macular anatomy (Fig. 8.6c–d) and RNFL thickness (Fig. 8.6e). Her vision improved to 20/25 OU within 6 weeks with only mild residual nasal disc edema OU.

Figure 8.7 shows a 22-year-old Caucasian female who presented with diplopia from a left 6th nerve palsy after snowboarding accident and was found to have a subdural hemorrhage causing increased intracranial pressure and papilledema. Her vision was 20/40 OU. Initial OCT (Fig. 8.7a) shows marked thickening of the peripapillary retinal nerve fiber layer. This edema extends beneath the retinal layers to produce subretinal fluid elevating the papillomacular

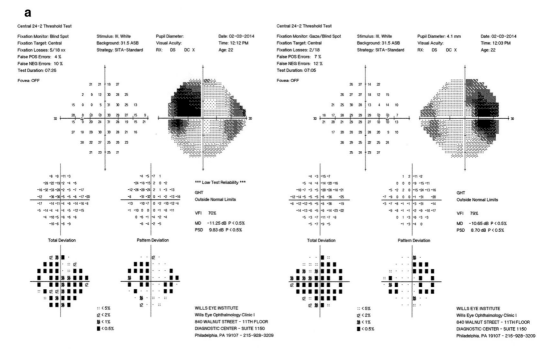

Fig. 8.6 Disc edema in pseudotumor cerebri. (**a**) Humphrey visual field on presentation showing enlargement of the blind spot in both eyes. (**b**) FoDi RNFL map of both eyes on presentation. Infrared image shows circumpapillary striae indicating subretinal fluid radiating from the optic nerve head toward the macula. Note that edema was so dramatic that the line tracing extends beyond the "above-normal thickness" portion of the chart. (**c**) Macular line scan of the right eye on presentation showing subretinal fluid migration into the foveola. The photoreceptors are disrupted, contributing to the 20/100 vision on presentation. The left eye appeared similar. (**d**) Macular line scan of the right eye on follow-up 6 weeks after initial presentation showing resolution of subretinal fluid in the macula. (**e**) FoDi RNFL map of both eyes on 2-week follow-up. Disc edema is resolving but still prominent

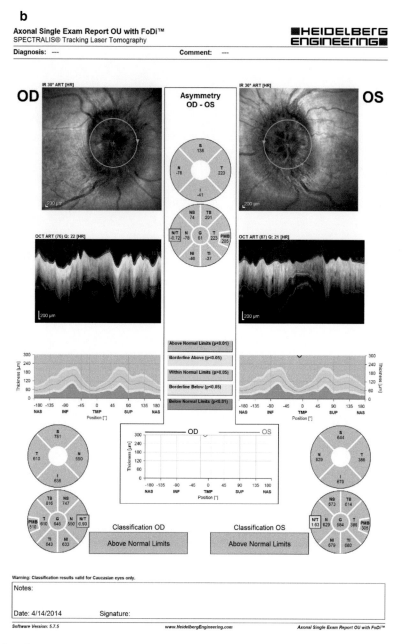

Fig. 8.6 (continued)

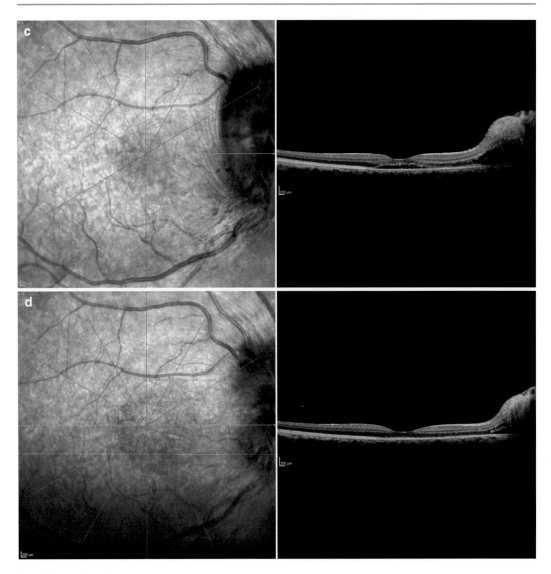

Fig. 8.6 (continued)

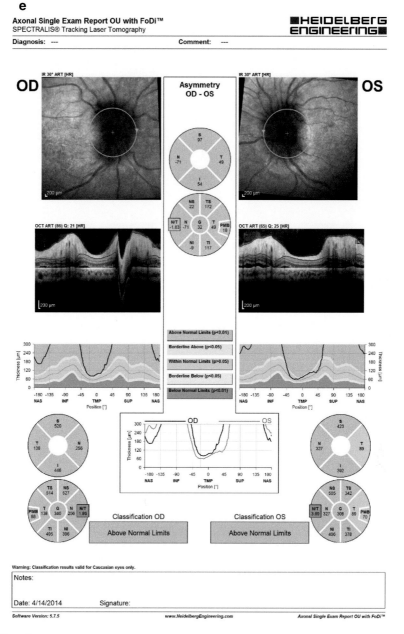

Fig. 8.6 (continued)

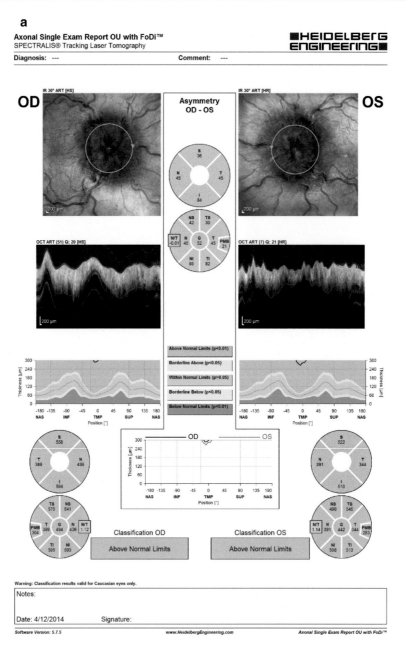

Fig. 8.7 Disc edema from subdural hemorrhage. (**a**) FoDi map showing bilateral disc edema on presentation with marked RNFL thickening in all quadrants. (**b**) Infrared image and macular line scan of the left eye showing marked subretinal fluid extending from the optic disc elevating the papillomacular bundle on presentation. Right eye appears similar. (**c**) *Vertical line* scan through the optic nerve head of the left eye on presentation, demonstrating the "lazy V" pattern of SHYPS [16]. The right eye was similar in appearance. (**d**) FoDi image showing 3-month follow-up of bilateral disc edema from elevated intracranial pressure. Note interval decrease in RNFL thickness, with residual edema bilaterally. (**e**) Macular line scan of the left eye showing near complete resolution of edema on 3-month follow-up. There are hyperreflective changes in the inner and outer plexiform layer near the optic disc. The right eye showed similar changes. (**f**) *Vertical line* scan through the optic nerve head of the left eye at 3-month follow-up demonstrating decreased but residual edema. Right eye was similar

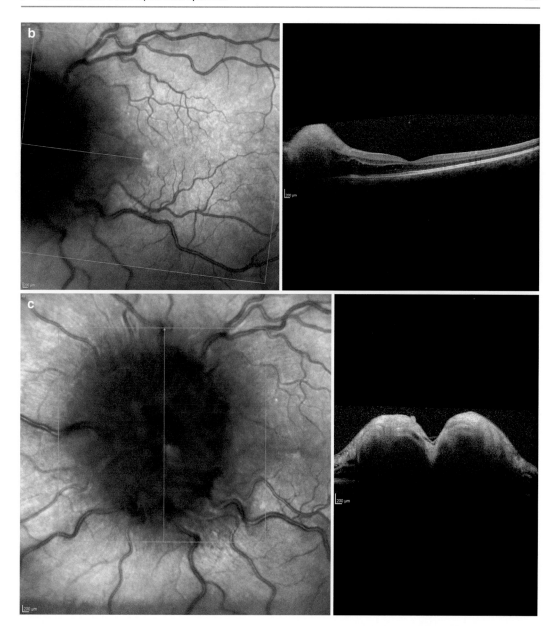

Fig. 8.7 (continued)

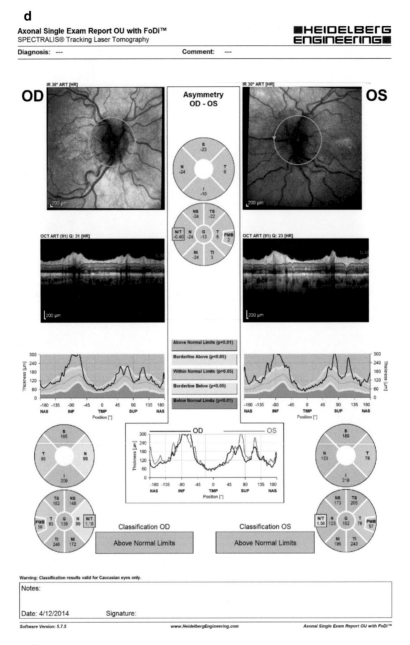

Fig. 8.7 (continued)

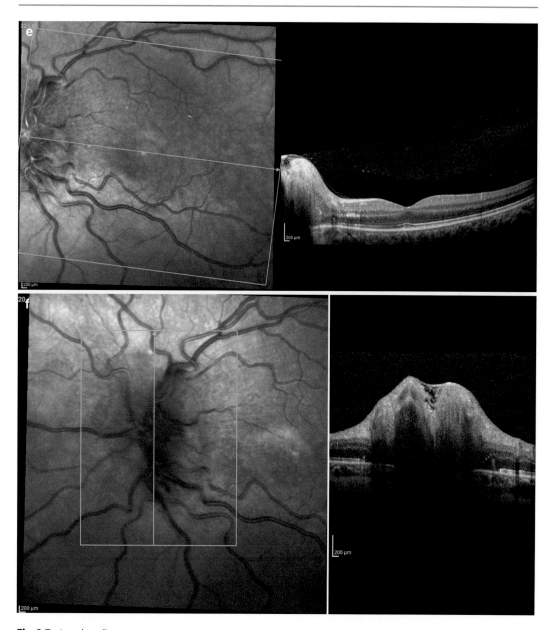

Fig. 8.7 (continued)

bundle (Fig. 8.7b). The "lazy V" pattern of the SHYPS [16] in disc edema can be seen on cross section of the optic nerve head (Fig. 8.7c). Three-month follow-up demonstrates improvement in peripapillary retinal nerve fiber layer thickness (Fig. 8.7d) and macular inner and outer segment changes in both eyes (Fig. 8.7e).

Anterior Ischemic Optic Neuropathy: NAION vs Giant Cell Arteritis

Nonarteritic Anterior Ischemic Optic Neuropathy

Nonarteritic anterior ischemic optic neuropathy (NAION) is, after glaucoma, the most common optic neuropathy in people older than age 50 with an incidence of approximately 0.5/100,000 for all ages and 2.3/100,000 for subjects 50 or older [17]. NAION classically presents with sudden, painless, unilateral vision loss with afferent papillary defect and inferior altitudinal field defect in a person over 50, usually discovered upon awakening in the morning. Nearly half of patients have visual acuity of ≥ 20/30 on presentation and one-quarter have vision ≤ 20/200 [18]. It is caused by ischemia of the anterior portion of the optic nerve head in the region of the lamina cribrosa and leads to segmental hyperemic disc edema, apoptosis of the retinal ganglion cell layer, and optic nerve atrophy with optic disc pallor by approximately 6 weeks [19, 20]. Risk factors can be divided into anatomic/ocular and systemic categories, and all available evidence indicates that the causes of NAION are multifactorial. Anatomic and ocular risk factors include "crowded" optic nerve (small or absent cup), optic disc drusen, cataract extraction, elevated intraocular pressure, and marked disc edema [21]. Systemic risk factors include diabetes, atherosclerosis ischemic heart disease, hypercholesterolemia, smoking, obstructive sleep apnea, systemic arterial hypertension, nocturnal arterial hypotension, migraine, and sildenafil (Viagra) use [21–25].

The pattern of damage of the retinal nerve fiber layer progresses from edema to loss over a 6-month period. Initial mean RNFL [19] thickness has been shown to be 189 ± 57 μm as compared to 96 ± 10 μm in normal eyes, progressing to 63 ± 14 μm at 6 months [26]. There does not appear to be further RNFL loss beyond the first 6 months, and any further thinning should prompt evaluation for alternate etiology of vision loss. Nerve fiber layer and ganglion cell losses have been shown to correlate well with visual field losses in magnitude and location [27]. Inferior altitudinal defects in visual field will therefore be reflected in corresponding superior retinal nerve fiber layer thinning and superior altitudinal ganglion cell layer loss [19, 27]. However, mean RNFL thickness in quadrants of the optic nerve head not corresponding to the visual field defects has also been shown to be significantly thinner when compared with uninvolved eyes, indicating damage beyond what is seen on visual field testing alone [19].

Figure 8.8 is from a 71-year-old female who had 2 months of visual disturbance in the left eye that she described as a grayish spot in her inferotemporal field of vision. Her visual field test revealed an inferior altitudinal defect in the left eye. Her vision was 20/200 OS with a 3+ relative afferent papillary defect. Her disc was noted to be pale, with resolving edema and papillary heme. The contralateral disc was noted to be crowded and anomalous. Initial RNFL scans showed normal RFNL thickness OD and increased RNFL thickness inferiorly and temporally OS (Fig. 8.8a). Her vision improved to 20/50 OS 5 months after the initial vision loss. ESR, CRP, and platelet counts were all normal. Her blood pressure was elevated at 190/90. Further questioning revealed a history of snoring and daytime fatigue, and a sleep study demonstrated severe obstructive sleep apnea. This revealed severe sleep apnea. Her blood pressure was controlled with oral medications. Follow-up OCT 6 weeks after the insult shows peripapillary retinal nerve fiber layer thinning (Fig. 8.8b) and interval macular thinning (Fig. 8.8c) consistent with an optic neuropathy.

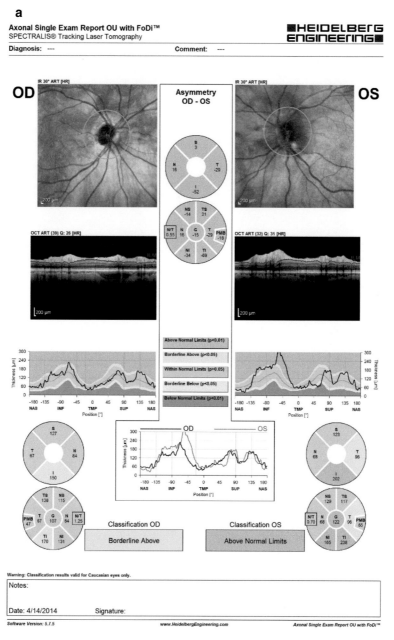

Fig. 8.8 Nonarteritic ischemic optic neuropathy. (**a**) Initial FoDi RNFL scans showing normal RNFL thickness OD and increased RNFL thickness inferiorly and temporally OS. Note the small and crowded optic nerve OD on the infrared image. (**b**) Six-week follow-up FoDi RNFL scan showing unchanged RFNL OD and RNFL thinning superiorly, temporally, and nasally OS. (**c**) Macular thickness map change report 6 weeks from baseline showing stable macular thickness OD and global macular thinning more pronounced near the papillomacular bundle and inferior fovea

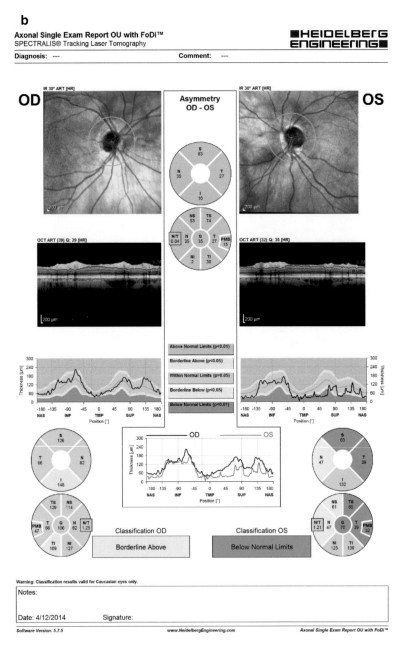

Fig. 8.8 (continued)

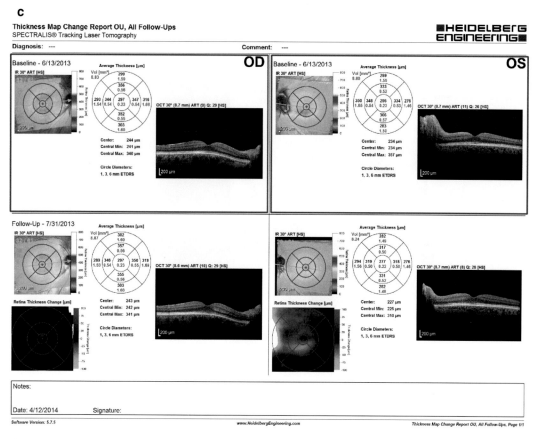

Fig. 8.8   (continued)

Arteritic Anterior Ischemic Optic Neuropathy: Giant Cell Arteritis

Although arteritic anterior ischemic optic neuropathy (AAION) is less common than NAION, this is an ocular emergency requiring early diagnosis and prompt treatment with systemic high-dose corticosteroids to prevent further visual loss. It is caused by inflammatory occlusion of the short posterior ciliary arteries and infarction of the optic nerve head producing pallid disc edema [22]. AAION occurs more commonly in women, and resulting vision is generally worse than NAION [28]. Symptoms suggestive of giant cell arteritis include headache, jaw claudication, weight loss, malaise, anorexia, and scalp tenderness.

Figure 8.9 is from a 70-year-old Caucasian female presented to the emergency room with a 1-week history of decreased vision in the inferior portion of her visual field. She had been feeling "flu-like" with headaches, scalp tenderness, and jaw claudication. Her vision on presentation was hand motions in the right eye and 20/30 in the left with reduced color plates and red and light desaturation in the right eye. The right optic nerve had segmental pallor nasally. Initial bloodwork revealed elevated platelets, erythrocyte sedimentation rate, and C-reactive protein. She was admitted for intravenous pulse corticosteroids and had a temporal artery biopsy that revealed inflammation of the internal elastic intima. Her symptoms responded to steroid therapy, though vision never improved beyond count fingers in the right eye. OCT on presentation (Fig. 8.9a) showed RNFL edema superiorly in the right eye. On follow-up 3 months later, OCT demonstrated superior, temporal, and nasal RNFL thinning OD (Fig. 8.9b).

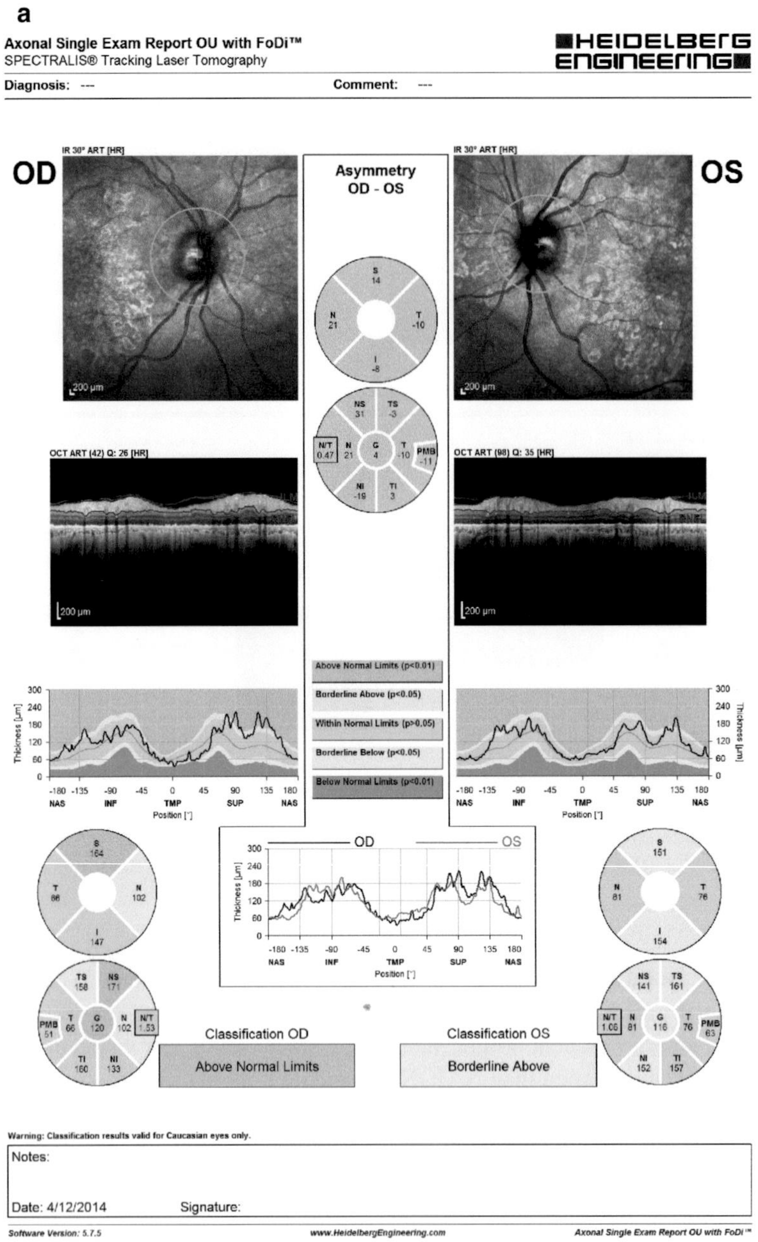

Fig. 8.9 Giant cell arteritis. (**a**) Initial FoDi RFNL map showing superior and borderline nasal RNFL thickening consistent with edema in the right eye. The left eye shows borderline thickening superiorly and inferiorly. (**b**) Three-month follow-up FoDi RNFL map shows superior, temporal, and borderline nasal thinning OD. The left eye is unchanged. Scattered areas of hyperreflectance on infrared image bilaterally are drusen from age-related macular degeneration. (**c**) Macular change map showing progressive RNFL loss in the right eye over 3 months as depicted by green coloration on the red-green map

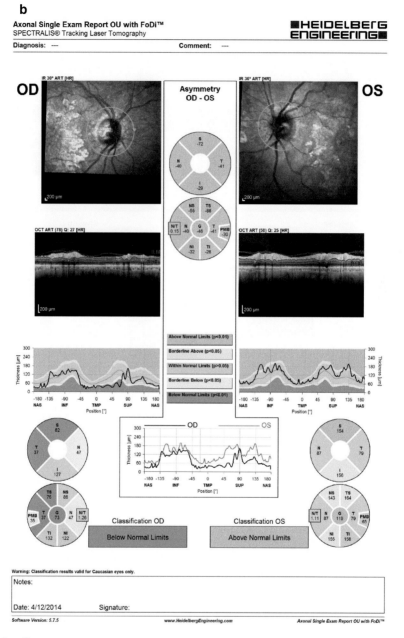

Fig. 8.9 (continued)

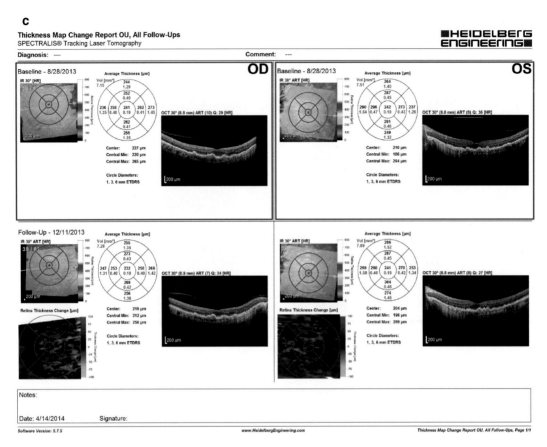

Fig. 8.9 (continued)

Figure 8.10 is from an 81-year-old Caucasian female who noted complete loss of vision in the right eye after 1 week of scalp pain and jaw claudication. On presentation to the emergency room, her vision was no light perception OD and 20/25 OS. ESR and CRP were both elevated. She was admitted for intravenous pulse steroids and transitioned to oral prednisone. Her ESR and CRP both normalized and the symptoms resolved. OCT imaging was obtained 7 months after initial presentation and showed dramatic RNFL loss OD (Fig. 8.10a) and macular RNFL asymmetry between the two eyes (Fig. 8.10b).

Optic Disc Drusen

Optic disc drusen are calcified prelaminar concretions of degenerated axonal tissue that occur in 0.3–2.4 % of the population and are bilateral in approximately 75 % of cases [29, 30]. They can be associated with visual field defects and ischemic optic neuropathy [31]. They can enlarge over time. Current methods of diagnosis include visualization on fundus exam, autofluorescence on fundus photography, and calcification on B-scan ultrasound or computed tomography. SD-OCT enables direct cross-sectional visualization of optic disc drusen at much higher resolution than that achievable using B-scan ultrasound or CT scan.

Differentiating optic disc drusen from true optic disc edema can be challenging [16]. The SHYPS (see section on Disc Edema, p. 124, for further explanation) has been noted to form a "lazy V" pattern in disc edema versus a "lumpy-bumpy" internal contour with abrupt decline in optic disc drusen [16]. Qualitative discrimination of optic disc drusen from disc edema based on OCT has been shown to have 63 % sensitivity

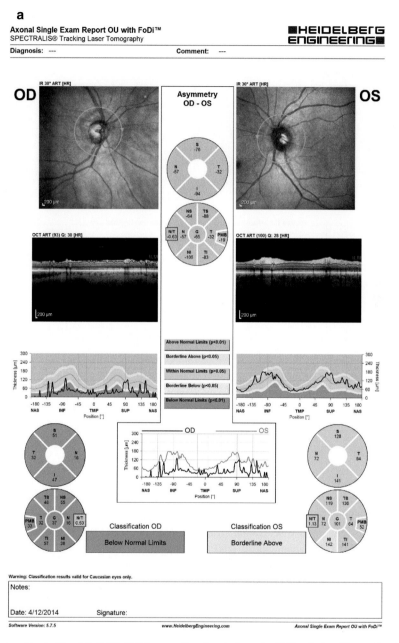

Fig. 8.10 Giant cell arteritis. (**a**) FoDi RNFL map 7 months after presentation showing near complete RNFL loss OD and normal RNFL OS. Note that the only spikes into the *green* normal values are in the areas of vascular bundles. Because both nasal and temporal RNFL are uni- formly lost, the N/T ratio is still considered normal. (**b**) Macular asymmetry map shows dramatic asymmetry between right and left eyes. The hemispheric asymmetry map shows greater inferior RNFL loss OD

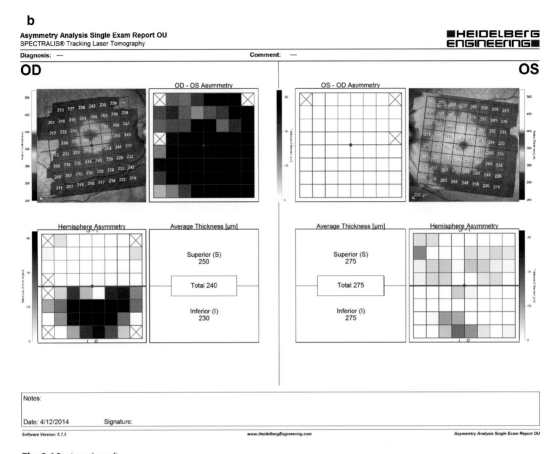

b

Asymmetry Analysis Single Exam Report OU
SPECTRALIS® Tracking Laser Tomography

■HEIDELBERG
ENGINEERING■

Fig. 8.10 (continued)

(true-positive rate) and 63 % specificity (true-negative rate), with most errors in diagnosis occurring distinguishing mild disc edema from subtle disc drusen [16]. However, nasal RNFL measurements have been shown to be significantly thinner for disc drusen than disc edema, bringing diagnostic sensitivity and specificity up to approximately 80 % and 70–89 %, respectively [16, 32].

Figure 8.11 is from a 24-year-old female who presented to the neuro-ophthalmology service with disc edema in both eyes. She had received an MRI and MRV which were both normal. Her optic discs were noted to be elevated without vessel obscurations. B-scan ultrasound showed calcifications at the optic nerve head bilaterally. Humphrey visual field testing was normal OD

and had possible paracentral changes OS. Fundus autofluorescence (Fig. 8.11c) showed bilateral hyperfluorescence, consistent with drusen formation.

Diabetic Papillopathy

Diabetic papillopathy is characterized by transient unilateral or bilateral optic disc swelling associated with minimal loss of vision. It can present with an approximately 0.5 % incidence in diabetics regardless of metabolic control or severity of diabetic retinopathy [33]. Disc swelling on clinical exam appears hyperemic and can last from 2 to 10 months with a mean duration of 3.7 months [33, 34]. The disc edema is often

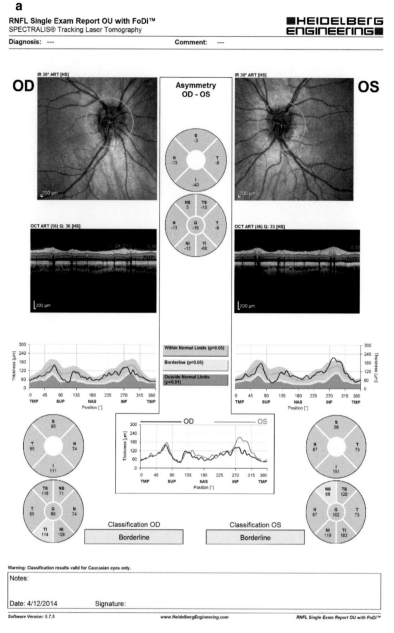

Fig. 8.11 Optic disc drusen. (**a**) FoDi map shows mild borderline bilateral superior thinning on the thickness tracings and mild borderline inferior thinning OD. These do not necessarily show up on the averaged thickness maps, and therefore interpretation of the *red-yellow-green* maps must be performed with caution. (**b**) *Horizontal line* scan with retinal thickness tracing of the right optic disc showing a characteristic "lumpy-bumpy" appearance for optic disc drusen. Note the absence of disc edema or fluid tracking into the surrounding peripapillary region. The left eye is similar in appearance. (**c**) Fundus autofluorescence demonstrating bilateral hyperfluorescence of the optic discs consistent with drusen formation

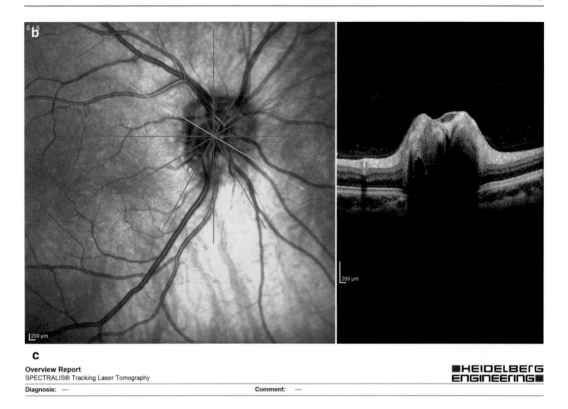

c
Overview Report
SPECTRALIS® Tracking Laser Tomography
HEIDELBERG ENGINEERING
Diagnosis: --- Comment: ---

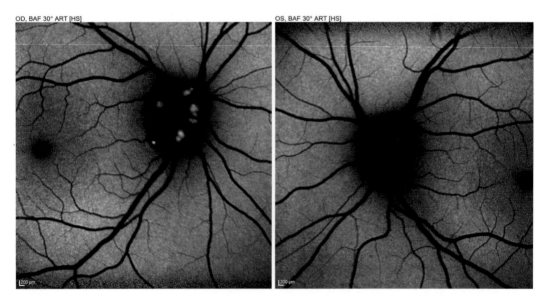

OD, BAF 30° ART [HS]   OS, BAF 30° ART [HS]

Notes:

Date: 4/14/2014   Signature:

Software Version: 5.7.5   www.HeidelbergEngineering.com   Overview Report, Page 1

Fig. 8.11 (continued)

accompanied by serous macular detachment causing decreased vision. Visual fields show a characteristic enlarged blind spot, as with other causes of disc edema. OCT findings include increased RNFL thickness and subretinal fluid seen on line scans.

Lyme Papillitis

Optic nerve involvement from the tick-borne spirochete *Borrelia burgdorferi* is a rare phenomenon, but is considered to be central nervous system infection requiring oral or parenteral antibiotic treatment [35]. Infection can cause bilateral papilledema from elevated intracranial pressure in children but rarely in adults. In adults, infection can rarely cause retrobulbar optic neuritis, neuroretinitis, and ischemic optic neuropathy. Workup for serum titers for Lyme antibodies should be included in any patient in a Lyme endemic area with optic neuritis.

References

1. Pasol J. Neuro-ophthalmic disease and optical coherence tomography: glaucoma look-alikes. Curr Opin Ophthalmol. 2011;22:124–32. doi:10.1097/ICU.0b013e328343c1a3.
2. Quigley HA. Neuronal death in glaucoma. Prog Retin Eye Res. 1999;18:39–57. doi:10.1016/S1350-9462(98)00014-7.
3. Sommer A, Katz J, Quigley HA, Miller NR, Robin AL, Richter RC, Witt KA. Clinically detectable nerve fiber atrophy precedes the onset of glaucomatous field loss. Arch Ophthalmol. 1991;109:77–83.
4. Lisboa R, Leite MT, Zangwill LM, Tafreshi A, Weinreb RN, Medeiros FA. Diagnosing preperimetric glaucoma with spectral domain optical coherence tomography. Ophthalmology. 2012;119:2261–9. doi:10.1016/j.ophtha.2012.06.009.
5. Nakatani Y, Higashide T, Ohkubo S, Takeda H, Sugiyama K. Evaluation of macular thickness and peripapillary retinal nerve fiber layer thickness for detection of early glaucoma using spectral domain optical coherence tomography. J Glaucoma. 2011;20:252–9. doi:10.1097/IJG.0b013e3181e079ed.
6. Zeimer R, Asrani S, Zou S, Quigley H, Jampel H. Quantitative detection of glaucomatous damage at the posterior pole by retinal thickness mapping. A pilot study. Ophthalmology. 1998;105:224–31.

7. Hood DC, Raza AS, de Moraes CGV, Liebmann JM, Ritch R. Glaucomatous damage of the macula. Prog Retin Eye Res. 2013;32:1–21. doi:10.1016/j.preteyeres.2012.08.003.
8. Greenfield DS. Macular thickness changes in glaucomatous optic neuropathy detected using optical coherence tomography. Arch Ophthalmol. 2003;121:41. doi:10.1001/archopht.121.1.41.
9. Hood DC, Kardon RH. A framework for comparing structural and functional measures of glaucomatous damage. Prog Retin Eye Res. 2007;26:688–710. doi:10.1016/j.preteyeres.2007.08.001.
10. Kanadani FN, Hood DC, Grippo TM, Wangsupadilok B, Harizman N, Greenstein VC, Liebmann JM, Ritch R. Structural and functional assessment of the macular region in patients with glaucoma. Br J Ophthalmol. 2006;90:1393–7. doi:10.1136/bjo.2006.099069.
11. Oberwahrenbrock T, Schippling S, Ringelstein M, Kaufhold F, Zimmermann H, Keser N, Young KL, Harmel J, Hartung H-P, Martin R, Paul F, Aktas O, Brandt AU. Retinal damage in multiple sclerosis disease subtypes measured by high-resolution optical coherence tomography. Mult Scler Int. 2012;2012:1–10. doi:10.1155/2012/530305.
12. Gordon-Lipkin E, Chodkowski B, Reich DS, Smith SA, Pulicken M, Balcer LJ, Frohman EM, Cutter G, Calabresi PA. Retinal nerve fiber layer is associated with brain atrophy in multiple sclerosis. Neurology. 2007;69:1603–9. doi:10.1212/01.wnl.0000295995.46586.ae.
13. Gelfand JM, Goodin DS, Boscardin WJ, Nolan R, Cuneo A, Green AJ. Retinal axonal loss begins early in the course of multiple sclerosis and is similar between progressive phenotypes. PLoS One. 2012;7, e36847. doi:10.1371/journal.pone.0036847.
14. Bichuetti DB, de Camargo AS, Falcão AB, Gonçalves FF, Tavares IM, de Oliveira EML. The retinal nerve fiber layer of patients with neuromyelitis optica and chronic relapsing optic neuritis is more severely damaged than patients with multiple sclerosis. J Neuroophthalmol. 2013;33:220–4. doi:10.1097/WNO.0b013e31829f39f1.
15. Sergott RC. Headaches associated with papilledema. Curr Pain Headache Rep. 2012;16:354–8. doi:10.1007/s11916-012-0283-x.
16. Johnson LN. Differentiating optic disc edema from optic nerve head drusen on optical coherence tomography. Arch Ophthalmol. 2009;127:45. doi:10.1001/archophthalmol.2008.524.
17. Johnson LN, Arnold AC. Incidence of nonarteritic and arteritic anterior ischemic optic neuropathy. Population-based study in the state of Missouri and Los Angeles County, California. J Neuroophthalmol Off J North Am Neuro Ophthalmol Soc. 1994;14:38–44.
18. Hayreh SS, Zimmerman MB. Nonarteritic anterior ischemic optic neuropathy. Ophthalmology. 2008;115:298–305.e2. doi:10.1016/j.ophtha.2007.05.027.
19. Dotan G, Goldstein M, Kesler A, Skarf B. Long-term retinal nerve fiber layer changes following nonarteritic

anterior ischemic optic neuropathy. Clin Ophthalmol. 2013;7:735–40. doi:10.2147/OPTH.S42522.

20. Levin LA. Apoptosis of retinal ganglion cells in anterior ischemic optic neuropathy. Arch Ophthalmol. 1996;114:488. doi:10.1001/archopht.1996.01100130484027.

21. Hayreh S. Management of ischemic optic neuropathies. Indian J Ophthalmol. 2011;59:123. doi:10.4103/0301-4738.77024.

22. Arnold AC. Pathogenesis of nonarteritic anterior ischemic optic neuropathy. J Neuroophthalmol Off J North Am Neuroophthalmol Soc. 2003;23:157–63.

23. Jacobson DM. Nonarteritic anterior ischemic optic neuropathy: a case-control study of potential risk factors. Arch Ophthalmol. 1997;115:1403. doi:10.1001/archopht.1997.01100160573008.

24. Mojon DS. Association between sleep apnea syndrome and nonarteritic anterior ischemic optic neuropathy. Arch Ophthalmol. 2002;120:601. doi:10.1001/archopht.120.5.601.

25. Pomeranz HD, Bhavsar AR. Nonarteritic ischemic optic neuropathy developing soon after use of sildenafil (viagra): a report of seven new cases. J Neuroophthalmol Off J North Am Neuroophthalmol Soc. 2005;25:9–13.

26. Bellusci C, Savini G, Carbonelli M, Carelli V, Sadun AA, Barboni P. Retinal nerve fiber layer thickness in nonarteritic anterior ischemic optic neuropathy: OCT characterization of the acute and resolving phases. Graefes Arch Clin Exp Ophthalmol. 2008;246:641–7. doi:10.1007/s00417-008-0767-x.

27. Aggarwal D, Tan O, Huang D, Sadun AA. Patterns of ganglion cell complex and nerve fiber layer loss in nonarteritic ischemic optic neuropathy by

fourier-domain optical coherence tomography. Invest Ophthalmol Vis Sci. 2012;53:4539–45. doi:10.1167/iovs.11-9300.

28. Danesh-Meyer HV, Boland MV, Savino PJ, Miller NR, Subramanian PS, Girkin CA, Quigley HA. Optic disc morphology in open-angle glaucoma compared with anterior ischemic optic neuropathies. Invest Ophthalmol Vis Sci. 2010;51:2003–10. doi:10.1167/iovs.09-3492.

29. Auw-Haedrich C, Staubach F, Witschel H. Optic disk drusen. Surv Ophthalmol. 2002;47:515–32. doi:10.1016/S0039-6257(02)00357-0.

30. Tso MO. Pathology and pathogenesis of drusen of the optic nervehead. Ophthalmology. 1981;88:1066–80.

31. Choi SS, Zawadzki RJ, Greiner MA, Werner JS, Keltner JL. Fourier-domain optical coherence tomography and adaptive optics reveal nerve fiber layer loss and photoreceptor changes in a patient with optic nerve drusen. J Neuroophthalmol. 2008;28:120–5. doi:10.1097/WNO.0b013e318175c6f5.

32. Lee KM, Woo SJ, Hwang J-M. Differentiation of optic nerve head drusen and optic disc edema with spectral-domain optical coherence tomography. Ophthalmology. 2011;118:971–7. doi:10.1016/j.ophtha.2010.09.006.

33. Regillo CD. Diabetic papillopathy: patient characteristics and fundus findings. Arch Ophthalmol. 1995;113:889. doi:10.1001/archopht.1995.01100070063026.

34. Nakamura M. Serous macular detachment due to diabetic papillopathy detected using optical coherence tomography. Arch Ophthalmol. 2009;127:105. doi:10.1001/archophthalmol.2008.533.

35. Träisk F, Lindquist L. Optic nerve involvement in Lyme disease. Curr Opin Ophthalmol. 2012;23:485–90. doi:10.1097/ICU.0b013e328358b1eb.

Index

A
Acquired retinal vascular diseases
  idiopathic macular telangiectasia, 56, 58
  Purtscher's retinopathy, 56, 57
  radiation retinopathy, 55–56
  RAM, 53, 55
  valsalva retinopathy, 57, 59
Acute posterior multifocal placoid pigment
      epitheliopathy (APMPPE)
  birdshot chorioretinopathy, 103–104
  symptoms, 103
  yellowish placoid lesions, 103
Age-related macular degeneration (ARMD)
  central visual acuity, loss of, 12
  exudative disease
    central choroidal neovascular membrane, 16, 21
    CNV, with retinal thickening and edema, 15, 18
    drusen and atrophy, 15, 19
    end-stage exudative ARMD, 15, 21
    large fibrovascular PED, 15, 16, 21, 22
    large hyperreflective sub-RPE membrane, 15, 18
    large PED, 15, 18, 19
    massive subfoveal choroidal neovascular
      membrane, 15, 19
    peripapillary choroidal neovascular membrane,
      15, 19
    post multiple anti-VEGF injections, 16, 22
    retinal hemorrhage, 15, 21
    severe exudative ARMD, 15, 16, 21
    topographic changes, 15, 19
  geographic atrophy
    bilateral, 14, 15
    central, 14, 16, 18
    disadvantages, 14
    macular atrophy, 14, 15
    nonexudative, 12, 13, 14
    superiority *vs.* modalities, 14, 17
  nongeographic atrophy, 12, 13
  prevalence, 12
Anterior ischemic optic neuropathy (AION)
  A-AION, 135–140
  NA-AION, 132–135
Anterior uveitis, 98, 99

Antivascular endothelial growth factor (VEGF)
    therapy, 12
ARMD. *See* Age-related macular degeneration (ARMD)
Arteritic anterior ischemic optic neuropathy (A-AION),
    135–140
Arteritic ischemic optic neuropathy (AION), 53

B
Birdshot chorioretinopathy, 103–104
Branch retinal artery occlusion (BRAO), 46–48
Branch retinal vein occlusion (BRVO), 41–42

C
Carboplatin, 85, 87
Cavernous hemangioma, 63, 64
Central retinal artery occlusion (CRAO), 48–49
Central retinal vein occlusion (CRVO), 44–47
Central serous chorioretinopathy (CSCR), 62
Choroidal hemangioma, 65,–66
Choroidal infarction, 50–51
Choroidal vascular diseases
  CSCR, 62
  PCV, 62–63
Cisplatin, 87
Clinically isolated syndrome (CIS), 115
CNS lymphoma, 107–108
Coats disease, 59, 61
Congenital retinal vascular diseases
  Coats disease, 59, 61
  FEVR, 58–59, 61
  ROP, 58, 60

D
Devic's disease. *See* Neuromyelitis optica (NMO)
Diabetic macular edema (DME)
  anti-vascular endothelial growth factor, 30, 35
  corticosteroid therapy, 30, 35
  with hyperreflective spots, 30, 32
  macular thickness mapping, 30, 32
  with nonproliferative diabetic retinopathy, 30, 31

© Springer International Publishing Switzerland 2016
A. Girach, R.C. Sergott (eds.), *Optical Coherence Tomography*,
DOI 10.1007/978-3-319-24817-2

Printed in the United States
By Bookmasters